From Scie

In From Scientist to Stroke Survivor: Life Redacted, Elly Katz creates a compelling, transcendent narrative of her experience as the survivor of a profound stroke. I strongly recommend this work for anyone engaged in the treatment or recovery process, whether as a medical professional, a caregiver, or a patient. Elly provides unique insight into the grief and pain of her experience while at the same time holding up a beacon of hope to anyone struggling to regain anything approaching "normalcy" after major injury or illness. This work combines poetry, testimony, and self-analysis to bring the reader into the world of someone experiencing life-altering change.

—Elena Kramer, Harvard University's Bussey Professor of
Organismic and Evolutionary Biology

Elly Katz has written a book about disability, about the loss and recovery of the physical and spiritual self, that it unlike anything I've read before. It's a profound and lyrical meditation on what it means to be alive, a book that will shatter your heart on one page and piece it back together on the next.

—Sam Apple, John's Hopkins Writing Program Coordinator and
Senior Lecturer in Writing

Elly Katz's From Scientist to Stroke Survivor-Life Redacted is a powerful look at trauma, disability, and the enduring power of the individual. This heart-wrenching and inspirational collection not only gives insight into the emotional toll of chronic disease and trauma, but what it is to be human—to more than persist, but to reconstruct after devastating loss.

I encourage anyone in the medical science community to read Elly's work as a way to better understand the human side of the ailments we study and aim to treat.

—Jenna Galloway, Associate Professor, Massachussets General Hospital and Harvard Medical School

From Scientist to Stroke Survivor: Life Redacted begins when Elly wakes up after a medical procedure and realizes something has profoundly changed. What follows is Elly's transformation; her transcendence into a new state of being.

Anyone who has experienced pain, loss—suffering that seems pointless—will benefit from this book. Pain, in this life, can be arbitrary and instantaneous. It can come from anywhere at any time. As Elly describes it, "Just as quickly as we enter the womb of the world, we can be pushed out, evaporated out of our current mentality and woken to hollow shells of ourselves."

Yet, out of loss sometimes comes a transcendence. Sometimes, loss is amplification—a direct line of sight without dilution. Elly writes for a simple reason: she has to. She writes because her soul is a percolating hotbox of raw feelings that needs to vent before it suffocates her. She writes to add edges to an amorphous future. This book is her gift to the world.

—Travis Christofferson, Author of Tripping Over the Truth

FROM SCIENTIST TO
STROKE SURVIVOR

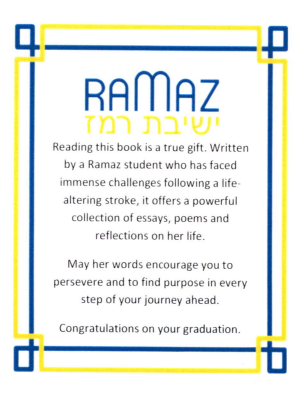

RAMAZ

ישיבת רמז

Reading this book is a true gift. Written
by a Ramaz student who has faced
immense challenges following a life-
altering stroke, it offers a powerful
collection of essays, poems and
reflections on her life.

May her words encourage you to
persevere and to find purpose in every
step of your journey ahead.

Congratulations on your graduation.

Elly Katz

FROM SCIENTIST TO STROKE SURVIVOR

Life Redacted

The Disability Studies Collection

Collection Editors

Damian Mellifont &
Jennifer Smith-Merry

To mom and dad
for meeting my metamorphoses—
my unmaking and my reinvention—
with profuse love.

First published in 2025 by Lived Places Publishing

The author and editors have made every effort to ensure the accuracy of information contained in this publication, but assume no responsibility for any errors, inaccuracies, inconsistencies, and omissions. Likewise, every effort has been made to contact copyright holders. If any copyright material has been reproduced unwittingly and without permission the Publisher will gladly receive information enabling them to rectify any error or omission in subsequent editions.

British Library Cataloguing in Publication Data
A CIP record for this book is available from the British Library

ISBN: 9781917503334 (pbk)
ISBN: 9781917503358 (ePDF)
ISBN: 9781917503341 (ePUB)

The right of Elly Katz to be identified as the Author of this work has been asserted by them in accordance with the Copyright, Design and Patents Act 1988.

Cover design by Fiachra McCarthy
Book design by Rachel Trolove of Twin Trail Design
Typeset by Newgen Publishing UK

Lived Places Publishing
P.O. Box 1845
47 Echo Avenue
Miller Place, NY 11764

www.livedplacespublishing.com

Bind me—I still can sing—
Banish—my mandolin
Strikes true within—

Slay—and my Soul shall rise
Chanting to Paradise—
Still thine.

—Emily Dickinson

Abstract

At age 27, working towards a PhD at Harvard Medical School, Elly went to a doctor for a mundane procedure to stabilize her neck. Her academic path was circuitous, its fits and starts an outgrowth of her connective tissue disease. That supposedly innocuous set of injections instantly transformed into a personal nightmare. Upon waking from anesthesia, she searched for the right half of her body, which she was unable to locate. Elly was rushed to intensive care in a state of limbo; her oxygen saturation nosedived, her heart slowed to a near stop, and numbness spilled from her spine throughout her right limbs. Somehow, she survived what doctors surmised was unsurvivable: a brainstem stroke secondary to a physician's needle misplacement. Her path towards a career in the sciences, among other ambitions in her life, came screeching to a halt.

As a devout writer, she feared poetry, too, fell outside her possible in light of her inert right fingers. But, in spite of this unfathomable plot-twist sustained at age 27, or, more aptly, because of it, Elly had to find a new mode of being. *From Scientist to Stroke Survivor: Life Redacted* is a creative account that enacts the nonlinear impact of trauma on the psyche. It poetically charts her zigzagging pilgrimage as she wrote through calamity to emergence.

Keywords

Trauma, Disability, Grief, Survival, Stroke, Surgery, Malpractice, Writing, Acceptance, Poetry, Creative Nonfiction, Scientist, Psyche, Mental Health, Art

Contents

Content warning

This collection of poetic nonfiction contains references to, and descriptions of, situations that may cause distress.

This includes:

- hospitalizations and medical settings
- descriptions of physical trauma and the subsequent rage, grief, physical and emotional pain, and despair that accompanied it

This is a story of disability and redemption. Please read with care.

Introduction

Since adolescence, Elly Katz was forced to acclimate to her health concerns. A connective tissue disorder, Ehlers-Danlos Syndrome (EDS), punctuated her high school and college years with interludes of illness in solitude, during which she developed a devotion to mathematics and science, sanctuaries of remediable variables. Elly's meandering path towards Harvard, and her seven-year journey into and out of its academic halls, fostered her scientific ambitions. Despite chronic pain, she interned in laboratories and ultimately earned admission to a doctorate in genetics.

In 2022, ongoing cervical instability, which is common in sufferers of EDS, convinced Elly to go to a doctor for a mundane, repeat set of injections. Anesthetized in the operating theatre, she was unconcerned; this exact procedure was familiar to her body. Waking on the other side of the procedure was a nightmare: a hemorrhage unleashed excruciating pain, and Elly searched in vain for her absent right half. The doctor's slip had caused a stroke.

Until tragedy flipped the script of her life, she assumed a stroke was something reserved for the old or decrepit, and its wreckage of the map of her body was unthinkable, impossible. She was met with doctors' incredulity at her survival against steeply stacked odds. However, she has survived. Since western medicine offered no salves to soften the blow to her brainstem, it has been up to Elly to engrave her own map, to define what it meant to endure her body's undoing. This collection is a testament to the experience of surviving the loss of one's body.

Learning objectives

At completion of this text, readers should be able to:

- become acquainted with the nonlinear experience of time in the wake of trauma, allowing them the opportunity to experience how trauma-survivors process the merging of their past into their present.

- identify how the speaker's description of experiences using poetic third-person narrative and her movement into and out of the past repeatedly stresses the disorienting force of grief in the recapitulation of sudden disability.

- experience the insistence of psychological dissonance that follows physical trauma, as well as the resulting isolation which complicates individual relationships.

- recognize the speaker's sense of shame, particularly the part played by ableist societal attitudes on that sense of shame.

- understand that an inability to overcome physical barriers doesn't imply a lack of resolve to endure them and make the best of obstacles.

- empathize with the frustration and anger due to an inability to get better, something which will, in time, help students be better practitioners if and when they work with individuals who have suffered physical, mental, and emotional traumas.

Part I
Overture

Her first experience was a penetrating itch. This sensation was layered on top of blistering pain shooting from the right part of her head into her eye. It was not the kind of feeling diminished by vigorous scratching, as is the case following a bug bite. Hers was a jaw-clenching urgency to dig her nails deeply into the right side of her scalp and face. She felt ignited, as if a vial of lightning was injected intravenously. It was all-consuming and unshakable, despite her clawing. Agony raged through her. The 1–10 subjective scale that doctors instructed her to rate pain stemming from her connective tissue disease recalibrated itself. Nothing could compete with this uproar—until the girl reckoned with her totalizing unanchoring.

Suddenly, she failed to locate her entire right side. The once watertight GPS system between her brain and her body was breached. "Mom, is my right side on the bed? Where is my right side? Can you see it? Is it there?" Her interrogatories gushed forth, the questions colliding with each other breathlessly as her terror mounted. Her throat constricted around syllables. Her body plan felt remapped to an uncharted terrain relative to before. This was after—the other side of wherever she had been, an elsewhere perpendicular to everything that framed her frameworks of time, space, herself and truth—she would not, could not, ever forget. It jolted her like a harrowing nightmare, a plot twist crafted in a science fiction workshop.

That is how traumatic cataclysms strike—in a slice of a second thrown off-balance. The world you assumed was a fixture turns out to be a balloon puncturable by a sharp blade. Paradoxically, the nervous system absorbs loss almost as gradually as it heals from an onslaught—gruelingly and ploddingly.

The sliver of a blessing inherent in this type of tragedy is the utter uncertainty, the absence of medical prognosis as to what may unfold in subsequent months and years. Sometimes, the unknown is what rescues. She is disoriented in her body. Everything the girl learned in Harvard's Evolutionary Biology lecture halls capsized internally. She felt herself in a state of decay as if she was a radioactive isotope leaking out of the lattice that held her universe up. Just as quickly as we enter the womb of the world, we can be pushed out, evaporated out of our current mentality, and woken to hollow shells of ourselves.

She could not determine where her right side ended, and the world began. Her sense of boundary dissolved. Her spine morphed from midline into a period, a hard stop, followed by a landslide of empty space. Her sense of center was catapulted to off-kilter. It still is. She lived out of context, at a remove from reference, inside the split-screen of her body. Her now overwrought and confused nervous system articulated a frightening fact. She forgot the geography of her right side, the drifting continents of ribs and limbs that were once paradoxically, disconcertingly, and lullingly welded to her torso. She could see it out of the periphery of her left eye. But feeling and seeing were so detached in her now. She longed to feel her right limbs against the gurney. She missed her once impervious right outline and felt like a vessel spilling out of herself, drop by drop, to the right.

Fear overtook her, gripping her in a chokehold, its sour taste festering on her tongue. Her mother stood beside her bearing witness, a mirror of dense horror. Despair pooled in both of their eyes. Silence enveloped them inside an igloo of trauma. Their mutual passion for language gave way to a stale quiet, an unfamiliar medium for both. They stared into the black abyss of immobilized space, endeavoring to divine something ineffable in the air.

Medical mishaps were part and parcel of what it meant to live in the girl's before body. Since age 8, hypermobility endowed her joints with too many degrees of freedom. She was always a step away from a kneecap or an arm dislocating. But the incidents she overcame with physical therapy were transitory. They did not etch themselves onto the pedestal of who she was and never jeopardized her potential. Now, for the first time, future and hope forsook her. An exotic vernacular of subtext—the semiotics of grimaces, winces, gasps, and glazed eyes—replaced vocabulary, too frictionless and blunt to express her baleful umbrage, her immanence in silence that left her mute. She felt unexpectedly atomized, cleared out of herself, by a tsunami.

The girl's goalposts disintegrated. She persisted at a peculiar angle in relation to the solid and resilient body that incurred routine subluxations but came through into new days unscathed, not permanently marked, disfigured, or disabled. She lived within the realm of risk yet within the vicinity of the mainstream, not in another solar system altogether.

She firmly shut and opened her eyelids while whispering prayers to a Judaic God she abandoned decades ago when her genetic connective tissue disorder, EDS, set in. In vain, she hoped that she was still in a daze from a cocktail of ketamine and propofol, that reality would kick in and the bilateral symmetry of the body she possessed prior to the doctor's near-fatal blunder would be restored. But there was no exit. There was no backpedaling into the person she was only three hours before. The physician who performed the procedure swiftly emerged by her bedside. He looked too debonair in his bespoke suit and necktie, as though he were ready for a party or a date in the direct aftermath of what would be his greatest medical malfeasance. Did he know? Did she? As he neared her, her inflection entered the highest register it does when her panic surges. "I can't feel anything on my right side. I can't move my right side. What's going on?" The words tumbled out of her. She did not have time for niceties. "Some of the local anesthetic probably tracked down your right side," he answered curtly. His tone was implacable. "You are fine and can go home," he advised as he ducked his head to look at an incoming text message. Much like his advent, he hurriedly departed the building, leaving the baffled girl and her mother in nurses' hands.

If you are wondering why she refers to herself in the third person, why this girl remains anonymous, it is because *she* no longer is— that person forever arrested in the ember, of Elly's, of my before. She glares at old photos of herself with accosting disgust. She simultaneously recognizes herself and does not. Her past could have been lifted off novel pages. My past.

I muddle and contuse pronouns over and again throughout this narrative, as I grapple with the lack of distance between me and myself. I write through and into an experience so massive that I require techniques to capture it. Poetry, in its permutations and repetition, is the one steadfast technology I leverage for this undertaking. I am not concerned with making meaning but with coming as close as possible to it. Therefore, the source of this artwork is a hovering presence; trauma's scale is a forest, while my ritual consists of drawing a single tree, a branch even, in lines of words that have proven to be essential lifelines. I glue myself together by taking a step back from the 'I', not to bypass it but to earn my right ultimately to occupy it again.

I am the ravages of what remains when the quotidian fades away. There is no path I can draw, no matter its digression or curvature, from here to there; there is but the bulwark we never sanction between before and after. Even as the body regresses, promulgating what feels like retrograde evolution, it is possible to pioneer an interior world. This is not, as you have likely gleaned, a strategic and methodological narrative. I have come to adopt the view that no life really fits that mold. This is not a valiant story of triumph over formidable adversity. Rather, it is a living document of learning to live beside my disability, and, intermittently, to even tap it on the shoulder, lock eyes with it and to feel worthy and robust in its precarious liminality.

She turned her back on her before, removing the Harvard degree that feels like a mockery from her wall. She fumes with ire at the brutal contrast between these two renditions of herself and wants to yell, to punch something, anything. She feels the sediment of this ghostly afterlife aggregating over her fossilizing self. Where did that girl participating in impassioned class discussions go? Recollections flood her. She feels like she is being waterboarded as trauma uncurls itself, its weeping wound reopening anew. But she will soon realize that forgetting is a more devastating anguish, a clamping down around the nebulous clouds of what peters out of awareness.

Almost two years later, she is sufficiently brazen enough to permit the old Elly out of the cage of her hippocampus every now and then, to let her walk about mental rooms and finger the wallpaper, as she sweeps through her deck of still-lives—the blonde mop of curls sparkling in summer racing against pink streamers fastened to her toddler bicycle, the scientist donning a pair of laboratory goggles, the girl sprawling across diagrams in mathematics textbooks as sleep caught her in the middle of homework.

No one warns you of the swift clip of tragedy, how you can blink and the tectonic plates of your universe rupture, swallowing you, dust particles discreetly falling out of the known world. She feels discombobulated and claustrophobic in the body she now shares with trauma. It feels too cramped for both of them. Her thoughts amass a surreal heft, a crushing gravity that threatens to break something in the brain that once made sense of everything. She has to set them down. Regenerative medicine was previously a wonder cure for her body, miraculously healing torn tendons and unstable joints from head to toe. Her succession of past successes with these interventions with the same doctor mollified any qualms about what should have been routine cervical injections, lending them the ease of stitches, or even of band-aid, removal.

We naturally other the infirmity we see in the world. We glance over and around wheelchair-bound individuals, ailments of the elderly, the blind reliant on walking sticks, limbs cast and dependent on crutches, and stroke survivors wearing distorted masks. A multitude of mental and physical disabilities are not even appraised by eyes curtly scanning, by minds concretizing a single thought into a myopic impression, because—like my connective tissue disease minus my stroke—these invisible impairments bluster below the skin and, therefore, are undermined, undervalued, and misapprehended. They are plagues, we convince ourselves, that cannot intercede in the zip code of our being, certainly outside the paved paradise of age 27. But no one is immune to inevitability; it can besiege anyone at any moment, irrespective of age. We are all closer than we can countenance losing our ways and our bodies.

That version of her **before October 24, 2022**—the day on which the threshold was erected between her and everything she thought iron-clad—will always be 27, preserved in the trap of recollection. Her former existence does not bear any resemblance to her now, a blip in the standard space-time continuum that runs at a remarkable delay, in which minutes feel like hours.

The narrow gates of disability are located elsewhere, an underground shadowland that only appears once you slip out of the socket of your ordinary, when you become a collage of machines and wires, your legs obsolete in the setting of your wheelchair, when your inner world stops spinning but the world outside continues to career about its axis, and when logic smacks against a monolith in the throes of unconscionable suffering. How blithely and all too casually it occurs, this machination of hurtling chance that sears you wide open.

Silence, darkness, and immobility—christening hallmarks of disability—befuddle the fortunate who fall somewhere within the statistical noise of the normal distribution. Disabled individuals are the unsung heroes of the unsung underworld. We hear but are unheard. We see but are not seen. We are phantoms. We are so real, so delicate and friable. Staring at our brokenness, our exoskeletons of bare mortality, it is like eyeballing Edvard Munch's *The Scream*—the yawning, agape mouth races through your bloodstream, a carnal and visceral repulsion ringing in your ears, until you glance in the opposite direction. It forces you to contend with too much humanity all at once.

The disabled do not have the luxury of swiveling their necks to face a diverting vista. If we could, we would hold ourselves at arms-length, create distance where there is only proximity. We want to bolt, to outmaneuver, to outsmart our circumstances, but where can we run when our feet can no longer carry us, when we aspire to outpace the heart thrumming within our very skin? We have nowhere to turn to but within—a secret door opening that was never tried. We are shoved off the conveyor belt of mundanity and become refugees out of place, incarcerated in bodies that no longer know our names.

She noticed she had to use the restroom. How does one sit up with half a body? For that matter, how does one do anything with half a body? The girl is still coming to terms with all of this. She is, almost two years later, asking the same question. She continues to receive silence in return. She is learning to dwell inside these questions. She no longer feels compelled to meet questions with prompt answers, as she did in Harvard math and genetics classrooms just a few months prior.

Against her will, she leaped from discerning genetic signatures of muscular dystrophy and spinal muscular atrophy to harboring her own rarer breed of disability she is, to this day, growing into. She treated neuroscience office hours like romantic encounters, the questions on action potentials whooshing through her, shooting stars illuminating the crisp sky of her intellect. After all, she has never been on a date, so how was she to know the difference?

She yearns for the sandpapered texture of knowledge, once an unassailable rubric, a hiding place she commandeered against the backdrop of chronic illness. She wrestles with her history in the gleeful throws of crafting a 300-page senior thesis on genetics, with the fact that she graduated Harvard *summa cum laude*. How and when did that all transpire? In her transfiguration into the present, she scrutinizes the thick red tape between chronic disease and her spinal cord stroke. How harsh and patent the segregation between her innocent before and this after.

She misses the truth of that girl who glistened at the crossroads of an equal sign of an equation, so accessible behind the covers of textbooks, beverages she gulped down in the form of mathematics solution sets running across reams of pages that never quite fit within the grip of the stapler. There was an unsullied and unspoken congruence between academia and veracity. Her potential, now barren and dejected, was then so sweeping and fertile, until it all fell apart.

She is astonished by her disappearance, a seeming feat of legerdemain—that girl who unabashedly flung her hand in the air in math lecture halls, gallivanted through science laboratories bursting at her seams with passion for the experiment she was about to conduct, and assiduously drafted papers in complex genetics classes. She was aloft on her own becoming and never felt the evanescence of being human, even in the face of her fragile connective tissue.

Her hobbies, plans, and blueprint were so immaculately laid out—the PhD program in genetics at Harvard Medical School she was asymptotically close to beginning and her ultimate dreams of a career in biotechnology. But that was derailed when the girl was curtained off from her known self, and obsolescence set in before her life even reached its midpoint. She witnessed ordinary sloth off its meaning, becoming a senseless string of sound. The disabled are scorched in the crossfire of a nuclear code set off in their very bodies. It's only now, two years since trauma took her hostage, that she is starting to adapt to her body's adaptation; it is only now that she is determined to endure. She is the victim. She is the evidence. She is the survivor. It is in her blood, her personhood, the caldron out of which she is gradually growing a new human she has yet to know.

She has been so mangled, externally and internally, that the doctor who violated her almost stole her name, which she nearly legally altered to Grace.

But her name, my name, holds my story. I am not willing to discard my past, even if it now feels like an item on recall.

All of this reeks of fantasy to her. He took it all. He keeps taking more from her with each passing day.

How he could, with the aid of imaging guidance that offered him direct eyesight into his target ligaments in her neck, pierce the girl's cervical cord and medulla remains an unanswerable question. He superimposed a spinal cord stroke and a brain hemorrhage on top of her already unstable neck and connective tissue.

Four nurses hoisted her up by her extremities and carried her to the adjacent bathroom. They did the same to bring her to her father's car. Her parents deduced that if they could safely drive home, as per the doctor's orders, then they could certainly bring their daughter to a trustworthy hospital adjacent to their apartment. Trepidation blotted out her rattling pain, whiting out the world—a shoreline from which she was washed away as she lay in the backseat.

Her body was an object now, but that did not, could not, concern her. She observed agitation stoke her parents, as though by osmosis they assimilated her own. Fraught wordlessness flossed through the car. None of the usual music played. Even the talking navigation system trailed off into silence. After all, what could language do in moments like these? Were there words for moments like these? She is still seeking them, as much as she is fighting to locate, to revive, her right side. She is learning the confines of language, the concept that because it is a human construct, it can only neatly contain other human constructs—linguistics, history, science, and other man-made disciplines—not the vagaries of happenstance. She is learning that oftentimes an absence of language is a word, that chasms can often cobweb more than meets the eye. She glances out of the window as nightfall skids across the horizon and her interior night begins to settle, a scar that may never fully heal.

She felt herself surrender to the tug at her very core as it snagged at the woman she presumed she was becoming. Instead of resisting the gravitational pull on her spirit, she let the heavy lethargy erupt inside her and embrace her like a weighted blanket strewn from anesthetic. She was at the mercy of the cosmos now, teetering on some precipice she could not yet call by name. She relented to the faint flicker of starlight, to the nearly inaudible tapping of her father's foot against the gas pedal, to her mother's cries escaping through the spaces between her fingertips—a maternal failure to blunt pain for her daughter's sake. She even yielded to her own brain, which felt as if it was disintegrating, crumbling like that blueberry muffin she consumed yesterday. Could that have only been yesterday? She could almost sense her neurons fragment into bits that could not, would not, ever again fire her into networks of completion. She reclined into the repose of memory, hazing into a trance. Inside her dreamscape, she tucked herself under the coverlet of the Memphis sky she imagined her ceiling to be as a child. All she felt was the loving roughness of her father's unshaven cheek brushing against her tender own.

But, without warning, her present began to rip and tear at the seams of her once indomitable fortress of childhood recollections, gnawing at the paneling of her naïveté. Her breaths grew shallow. She panted, as though suffocating under the vortex of a riptide, the water spinning her into a dizzying tailspin beneath its bottomless depths. The wrenching, stabbing pain in her right scalp drowned out all else, even the lack of sensation from the right side of her neck down that half of her body. Who knew that numbness itself was a feeling, a hostile intensity?

She capitulated to it all—to the body that was no longer hers, to the soul that may be in partial flight to another habitat, to the presence and absence of everything she felt and could not feel. She let herself melt into the car's to-and-fro as traffic hissed and wheezed them towards the emergency room of a Manhattan hospital. She could sense herself unspooling. The edges of the world were pressing in on her from all sides as her body was manhandled onto a gurney and into the scanner that would bracket and barb the rest of her life.

An urgent question bounced off the walls of the CT scanning room, a refrain dripping with untamed concern. "Is my right side on the table?" Her voice did not sound like hers. It had an infantile and a near-tearful quality. It sounded so foreign to her that she shifted her gaze about the room for its owner. At age 27, she was accustomed to her maturing, almost raspy, voice. She adored her deliberate pace of speech as she selected words as though they were books at a store, testing out vocabulary as she did initial paragraphs on for size inside her brain before committing to a given set of syllables or a novel. But she did not have that aptitude now. Ironically, she was held captive and still within her body, but her brain was on overdrive, running at a fast clip to make sense of her biological collapse. The words poured through her lips in a torrent, one bleeding into the next as though a paucity in the space-time spectrum was setting in, as though the laws of quantum mechanics could be subverted.

Her memories feel blurry since that instant, since that question, which would become her newfound chorus line, skipped through the air, more like jagged pieces than anything coherent, desecrated like her spinal cord and brainstem. She recalls the traces of her parents' tears as her gurney exited the exam room, the worry stitching into and smudging their expressions into hodgepodges of wrinkled skin and coiled muscles. She remembers the cool wisps of air entering her nostrils as a nasal cannula was inserted and hands wheeled her into intensive care.

But there is one moment, or rather, a string of moments, that shine through the cracks in her mind, a light radiating the nightmarish black clouding that time. Her mother is in a chair beside her and cradles her daughter's left hand, the sole hand she can feel. The girl knows she is a planet and a half from alright. She does not need to hear it to know it. The words are plainly stenciled onto her mother's anguished countenance. "Mom, let me have a bite of the peanut butter sandwich," the girl requests even though she's been told not to consume anything in case emergent surgery is needed. "We can't. I wish I could give it to you," the mother is aggrieved by this measly disappointment. But, if she is honest, she is devastated by its subliminal connotation—about all of the "no's" that will forever present themselves to her now disabled daughter, about beginning this solemn track record for her girl. She knows she is doing the right thing but dreads the message she relays. "Please Mom, I promise not to say a thing if you don't. This may be the last bite of food I ever eat." This is when the mother uncontrollably cries before her daughter, who is keenly aware that she may be in the final period of her life.

They both know this exchange could be their curtain call. The mother relents and passes her daughter the sandwich, as she quickly scans past the glass door to ensure no doctor is within eyesight. They laugh and cry and laugh again. This is an episode they cannot ever forget. While the girl comes unglued, her unity with her mother is unbreakable, firmly tethered to something that surpasses her downtrodden body, that supersedes anything and everything on Earth. The girl will soon concede that neither knowledge nor education will pull her through this bleak quicksand, that her one true constant in this world is the woman looking back at her and smiling through tears.

The medulla, an inherited swath of the reptilian brain, is a critical but overlooked component of our nature. Located at the base of the skull, it is the seat of our primordial impulses—the control panel of hunger, thirst, respiration, oxygenation, heart rate, and urination, among other basic inclinations.

The doctor's malpractice needled into my medulla the recrudescing question of what it means to be a human being deprived of human instincts. I miss the empty feelings of hunger and thirst, absences only felt in their absolute absence. I am barred from recovery, my being subscribed indefinitely to ambiguity, to the drunken turtle pace of the central nervous system's faltering but dogged yearning to heal. Some wounds overrun the brilliance of the body.

My medullary stroke also altered the once beautiful dynamic between my heart rhythm and oxygen saturation, which now engage in a vertiginous see-saw with each other that almost removed me from this world. When my grief soars, I compel myself to remember how fortunate I was to land in this limbo, how a fraction of a millimeter could have inverted my outcome— the frightening tug-of-war between life and death that played out during my stint in intensive care.

My survival imparts me the tenacity to design my world anew with genuine sincerity. The intensive care ward battered me into the artistry of doing more with less, a remarkably arduous lesson given the rigidity I imposed on my world under the dazzling false premise that I could author the arc of my life, that life follows an arc at all.

Now, in the aftermath of this insult to my brainstem, I am dependent on external oxygen delivered via nasal cannula. I am humiliated before my mother, who only greets my divested body with an abundance of fierce love. Her forbearance with me catches fire somewhere deep within, inducing me to begin to find nuanced enchantment in this vulnerability, to whisper to myself a less horrific healing story, to acclimate to hope's new configuration, to pinpoint it and to begin to quest for what can be hoped for when the woman you invested 27 years in becoming no longer exists. My mother renegotiates the terms of my destruction in her quiet position beside me, her tender palm between my shoulder blades, a poem of touch sheathed in a benediction. This is our downsized, revised version of a hug, a caress that talks me out of my own emptiness. This gesture feels like Earth is sighing after holding its breath, awaiting an end to this after that does not arrive.

"Mom," I hissed the other night as we pantomimed our bedtime ritual, "remember that potty-training book with the red plastic cover you read to me as a child?" My gloom cracked, forfeiting to a vitalizing bit of sarcasm. "Yeah, Bel. Why?" My mother's sheepish eyes blinked into the glistening tracks of my tears. Night crested in shadowy waves through my bedroom. "I think I am now reading that book backwards, reverse engineering myself. I am literally defying evolution. Darwin would be inconsolable." I crouched my spine as I spoke, my whisper snapping with sardonic levity, the convexity of my body emulating its internal fissures. But our eyes converged again, and I found belonging in my mother's blue irises swimming with sadness tinged with the joy that I could still insert humor into encounters like these.

I can no longer keep up with my contemporaries, with New York City or with myself. But I refuse to give myself back to the stardust from which I came. I am not ready yet. I am not done yet. But, in order to contend with my current draft of existence, I often need to role-play as the observer, pretending there is some dystopian farce underway—that none of this is as definitive or delineating as it actually is.

During my eight-week inpatient stay, time developed an elasticity I would grow into, its intervals stretching into expandable wads of chewing gum. My anguish and loss seemed to dismantle everything, distending time, rendering it too taxing for minutes to carry on at their typical clip.

However, I was not alone. My parents became abiding pillars of steel. I knew and felt their unflinching allegiance prior to this tragedy but had never tested and measured the extraordinary lengths to which they would go to be with me during this try-ing course. They modify reality to every extent possible as it uncorks before me so I can withstand the suffering that never stops. Instead of changing my name to Grace, I opted to find the grace in still being Elly. A year later, I decided that the doctor who malmed me plundered enough. I am still fighting an uphill battle and refuse to give up on life because of their refusal to give up on me.

For the duration of our time at the hospital, my father slept upright in a plastic chair, affording my mother the only slightly more comfortable recliner. He captured levity just as he once educated me to ensnare the rare lightning bugs in Tennessee, prudently opening and tightly closing the lid of a jar to maximize the insects' longevity.

Each night, I took inventory of my right side with my left hand, groping until skin met other skin that felt like rubber, not any-thing corporeal. I am still on that same sensory treasure hunt for the half of me that resides in some subterranean basement of my nervous system. I am indefatigable in my futile effort to coax feeling back into the jumble of limbs I forget and remember, a broken record cutting into and out of consciousness. I dread the darkness of nighttime most; at least in daylight, I can see my right leg, arm, and torso and consider myself somewhat unified. In the darkest dark, the laxity of nostalgia tugs and tugs, a rope encircling my ankles, lurching me into ever-deepening waters of ruminative mourning.

The attending's pronouncement of the paralysis of my right half, fortunately, was expunged by movement's jerky crawl back into my right extremities, deserts of awareness. A unilateral corridor opened between my eyes and my right limbs, an unspoken discourse of motion that, more often than not, produces a chaotic frenzy of involuntary movements. My arm skyrockets through the atmosphere landing overhead, or behind my back, as I grasp for it, an anxious game of hide and seek. Other than my twisted visual field, another ongoing symptom of my bewildered medulla, the closest thing I have to a tracking device for my right arm is my mother. I awaken into twilight and bellow into the intercom system joining my bedroom to that of my parents for my mother. I seethe with maddening rage as I falter to feel my path with my left palm to my right arm, which is frequently dislocated overhead. I spend outrageously up to 40 percent of a day eyeing and babysitting my limbs, an ongoing dynamic of *Where Is Waldo?*.

The vacuum of sensation and joint awareness on my right side leads my right arm and leg to become staggering deadweights that heave and pull on my body, manacles of unwieldy heaviness that feel more like the state of Texas than body parts. I am fastened to tunneling emptiness, a gnawing hunger or thirst, biological networks profoundly missed, that disorganizes and deconstructs thoughts.

It took me a month to navigate from my bedside to the com- mode, to stand but for a brief instant on a leg that was not, could not, belong to me. I feel like I free-fall onto air each time my right foot strikes ground. I spent the majority of that bed-bound hos- pitalization letting minutes tick by, hoping I could somehow trick them with my once brilliant mind into squinting into the brevity of seconds I had known so well, wishing for them to glide over me like tap water over hands.

If losses were a currency, I am convinced I could purchase any- thing. My right ear no longer hears the world but has become decorative. I cannot taste nor sense food in the right side of my mouth. I am deleted of depth perception and right periph- eral vision, which has collapsed reality into a flatland inside my defective brain. The irony hits me like a brutal slap across the cheek that in losing physical perspective—paramount to the physics and math once a mainstay in my life—my mental land- scape arborized, arraying too much resonance about mortality, meaning and heartbreak. All this cemented over my already vast knowledge base that commenced its growth-spurt when chronic illness, in the form of EDS, took hold. I did not brush my right teeth for eight months, because those teeth neglected to notify me of their continuous existence. Thankfully, a mirror quickly course-corrected the downward trajectory of my forgot- ten enamel. I cannot perceive my entire right half, aside from electric agony stinging my head—my brain bleed's footprint on my cranial nerves—and nerve pain that seethes across my chest and rib cage from my daily overdose of dislocations.

And what have I gained? Vestibular symptoms that render me forever spinning in the teacups on Coney Island, perennially on the verge of choking on my gastric acid and paresthesia—involuntary muscle contractions that cause my right limbs to flail about of their own accord and feel like micro-seizures rinsing through my right side. Imagine what it would feel like if every cell on one side of your body was converted into a vibrating cell phone. That is how I experience the world. Nothing staves off these persistent effects.

I wrote myself out of my family, incentivized by my incompetence to perform any task, however simple, on my own at age 27. I could not rekindle the student who feasted on spurious correlations and clung to extrinsic validation, the alleged meritocracy of academia. So, I hunkered down in the bunker of my bedroom. But, to my dismay, the world found me over and again in a whiplash of emails from professors and friends eager to know what I was up to, how my doctoral studies were progressing or if I was flirting with any romantic relationships. These unanswered correspondences felt like car crashes that upended thought processes. I wept and screamed until enervation gave way to sleep. My survival could not occur in seclusion, because the modern world had, gallingly, not been overturned by my stroke. A significant portion of me, at age 29, is grateful for that fact—for the tablet on which I now make words meet, participate in online yoga classes and listen to poetry. Technology is the vehicle through which I evacuate my body and enter the safety-net of belonging. Yet, the cost is unremitting. Before, I was a 27-year-old sometimes inept in distinguishing left from right. Now, I am an expert in that regard. In this after, I stuttered over who I was and desired to renew my lease on the girl who slaved with alacrity over her GPA and mistook empirical formulas for planetary gears. I thought I could calculate my way into a pres-aged future consisting of boyfriends, a nuclear family of my own, a scientific career, and a myriad of sacrosanct trivial experiences discharged of instantaneous hardships that prodded me out of my familiar. Who are you when all of your defining attributes are erased, save for in the biting stretch of memory? Life torn at its seams. Meaning seemed to decode its way out of my creation. I was amorphous, my right limbs adrift in the translation of my trespassed nervous system.

I felt like a lightning rod. My brothers' job prospects and expand-ing families became the lightning that zapped the relative grim tempest of my body. I was excessively sensitized. Existence became a tolerance challenge. My stamina circled the drain. My envy of my brothers' lives fed my sense of unworthiness of being cherished in this wasteland. I sorely stepped over the insight that there is no premise, no precondition, their love stipulates. It is an unalloyed element unexamined on the periodic table. But, in the muck of my sadness, I built a dam against the tides of my nieces' footfalls on floorboards and my nephew's laughter beyond my bedroom. For roughly a year and a half, the guiding motif in my life was to keep myself secreted away, incognito. From my van-tage point behind the camera lens of reality—at once painfully close and impossibly remote from the shores of my possible—I thirsted for occupation—to catalyze one more laboratory reac-tion, to solve one more derivative. I was embarrassed, impatient, and uncomfortable with myself. I fruitlessly aimed to defer life until I became fluent in the vocabulary of my right side. Now, instead of frustrating me endlessly, my right half beguiles me with a desire to know it with the wisdom that such knowing may not be part of my future.

Almost two years since my body hit the landmine of my stroke, I am revising how I live in this body. My mind alights on what persists. I am learning that the wall between my before and after is, actually, a dotted line rather than anything solid, more penetrable than impassible. While the doctor's needle distorted and disrupted my right half, it distresses me to admit that I neglected the toll that same misstep exacted on my immediate family—once invincible and now overcast with a trillion invisible fracture lines.

I am adapting to my shadow. I am rebooting myself. I am discovering that I am mutable, that there are components of my narrative I can include or exclude. I recognize that while the doctor pruned central neurons and synapses in my nervous system, I, not he, unwittingly, pruned my own siblings out of my life. But my brothers were permeable ions ready to migrate into me after the whole time. They held fast to that inkling, even when it rebounded off my consciousness for too long.

It dawned on me only recently that I do not need to muffle their happiness, that it is deeply unfair and unfortunate of me to project their blossoming existences onto the prism of what my life now lacks. As I wake into this revelation, I crave to simply be in their presence without scouring for words that will never encapsulate the love we share. I do not know if I will ever be capable of repaying the debt of their patience with me as I begin to settle into disability. I do not know if they even require retribution, other than my acceptance of them and their children, despite my epic failure to accept my faulty body. Now, I feel indescribably blessed for their return into my bedroom, for time shared in silence, for the gift of interdigitating my fingers into my brother's open palm. I feel less flustered, less redacted, when I am in my brothers' company, when our eyes engage in unspoken conversation. I now hug my nieces and nephew with my left arm, holding them as they steady me, educating me never to let go again.

This sea-change in what I can still control in this wallowing body does not imply that my grief has achieved closure. Rather, I volley back and forth between hiring myself and retiring from the project of my body at least twice a day. I often feel debased, but I intuit a juncture between extermination and evolution and aspire to drive my way into transformation. In that vein, I am reaching towards my brothers and their children, weaving them into my incredibly mortal world, so that I am rooted in what is, what was, and what will always be, no matter how my body behaves.

The combination of my connective tissue disorder and this injury has drastically altered my right side—a blood-crusted text of trauma scarred from migrations of ribs and limbs out of the socket. Even my dreams are tainted and hazardous. The puzzle of my body perched on nighttime falls into disrepair upon waking. The breaths of courage I summon are often inadequate. I am concussed over and again with just how broken I am, the pace at which trauma dispassionately taunts the mind with cognitive dissonance.

I undertake the massive architectural project of my body each day by staring my way into a mirror, into body parts on my right-side starving for sensation, as I dictate into my phone precisely which ribs and limbs have transgressed their boundaries and the angles at which I find them. I spend two to three hours reconstructing and stabilizing my perplexing form and realize the sorrowful yet triumphant insight that this is my 29-year-old version of independence, that the endurance of my body and soul can never be recanted because I survived what should have been the unsurvivable. Oftentimes, my glance swipes across my face, and I see in my eyes something at once familiar and strange, someone inescapably mortal and shattered. I feel disjointed from my former life, uncertain how I landed here, looking for a through-line yoking my before and after that does not exist. Then, my eyes ping to the illustration on my wall of neurons emblazoned with the word "survivor" in chalky letters. I feel a quickening of my own throbbing pulse, the seed of belief in a beginning taking root.

Now, as I look my way into my being, I witness someone who does not want to resist a right side no longer leashed to her brain, someone who does not want to hurt herself more than she has been hurt, someone who views the long stretch of her shadow as the elegant child of darkness and light, someone for whom the words tomorrow and walk feel like electrocution from within, but someone who is unveiling the discipline of gardening her soul born of the infinite time and finite space of disability. I will always long for that girl I once was wandering through the loom of Cambridge side streets, elbow locked in that of a friend while discussing firing patterns of neurons and how they appeared like Van Gogh's *Starry Night*. I consistently receive somatic reminders that I am, that all of us are a work of art.

But blinding sunsets liberating the clot of darkness, thoughts of dolphins dancing through frosted ocean waves, symphonies of rain kissing windows, jazz ensembles that rock me from within with emotion, escape hatches of majestic literature, birds chirping in blistering winter, the fertility of soil rippling through land, wind running through trees and spellbinding mountains situated between Earth and heaven—oh, there is yet endless beauty to behold in this broken world, in this derailed life, in this catastrophic body.

I must reflect on the small but mighty graces that accompany my apocalypse. The hushed humming through my right interior—I yearn to know you, darling right side—you and I are torn asunder, but undeniably alive in this aftermath. An about-face of consciousness is taking hold, prompting me to quit my deluded post in the Grand Central Terminal of my brain and to practice listening intently to my body. I am a process, unfinished and unfinishable. We all are. I hope this impresses upon you how incalculably precious you are, irrespective of the state of your physical constitution.

Each night, my father filibusters for my innocence. My frosted eyes thaw as we toss laughter back and forth at our living non-sequitur. He relinquishes his phone, the tail-end of his workday, social obligations, or anything else for a partial smile to brush across my face, for quixotic glee to flicker in my eyes. He creates what feels like a commodious space within the narrow corridors of disability, in which he and my mother live with me, a triad that shares the burden of my loss.

We no longer reach into the pockets of planners or calendars— relics from another lifetime—but linger in the now. Just as abruptly as it was washed away, my naïveté courses through my shipwrecked body in absurd laughter at the outrageous mayhem of our days, keenly honed into my father's witty banter with me as he pushes me in my wheelchair from kitchen to bedroom, sanctifying me with his jocularity into everything and nothing, the question drizzling with tragicomedy of what vacation means anymore in the sling of our surreal reality.

We become something verging on one entwined entity in my bedroom as the dark night finds us. My mother's voice, smothered by the syncopated whining hiss of my oxygen concentrator, becomes a static footprint of high pitch. I hear my father's smirk, the glint in his eyes, when he says, "Karin, why don't you go into a room even further away, so we can't hear you a bit better." From her dominion at her computer several rooms away from us, my mother doesn't hear his reply. But that's beside his target point. My father is entertaining me, indulging me in the humor of his words. He leans over my resting body, holding an iPad overhead, an adult dreamcatcher in my father's hands, at the precise angle I need to see it. We watch Ray Charles' unparalleled performance of "Song for You" liberating so much feeling. We listen and sing along to Eric Clapton's "Running on Faith", the words continually getting caught on dropped stitches of my soul. We can almost touch the lyrics. They are that real. My father is my remarkable cultural liaison, my gateway into a forbidden world that ruptured at my feet.

My once-ample energy generator dwindled in the bruise inside my brain, and I dumped the remainder into anger and resentment so lava hot that I could sense my cheeks grow beet red, tension wire lines across my forehead and into my jaw—at this derangement from self, at the rapacious doctor who flung me out of my own form. My world became one of austere sharp corners. I was thrown out of linearity, out of sync with the world, on some intergalactic space shuttle meandering to another universe. Even syllables are no longer integrated into sense. The world was a cruel mutiny, a museum out of bounds. I felt terrorized by my story. I fretted. I itched to relent. After eight mentally abusive months, I decided that courage was something ripe I could pluck. It dawned on me that how I tell my story was, unlike its thorny facts, up to me. My oxygen-depleted brain was kinked, a seemingly useless organ no longer treading thoughts that once marathoned through me in linear algebra lectures.

I regained the leisure of digesting literature within the overground tunnel of the hyperbaric chamber, a sealed cylinder of pressurized oxygen readily accessible to my bloodstream. I now knock on doors of terse marvelous verses that diminish my loneliness, connect me to what feels like the entire galaxy. The physical synapse decimated by the doctor's blade was replaced by more a subtle synapse, a webbing between me and other authors. David Whyte, Marie Howe, Ada Limón, Emily Dickinson, T.S. Eliot, among other voices, cut into me bloodlessly, poetry that rattles through me with gilded luminosity. I listen to their mellifluous work as my socked feet dance on the walls of the chamber. Riffs of rhythm and meter perfume the silence, notes shimmering in the air. I am struck by an epiphany that the decadent taste of faith shaped into words was not hijacked by my stroke. Their language reinstates my incorrigible obsession with the written word, repatriates me into chains of syllables. I view poetry as an internal audit, a means of feeling my way into this stormed body.

I have hesitantly and slowly found the pen inside my vocal cords, the means by which I am dictating my way into this sentence. Life is inside out, flipped, but I am leaning into being on the cracked streets of this body, this disabled species of existence, forging my own legacy without an itinerary. I still feel inarguably regressive, torn like a magazine article out of my life. I refuse to regurgitate my unmaking in plain language, to lend it another life in my mind. But, as a writer, I am propelled to create and could not write about anything other than this untemplated side of being, a lion roaring ceaselessly in my ears. So, I turned to poetry, a verbal indirect attack through scenic tributaries of metaphor, not the pointed, unpolished truth of prose. At our essences, we are all poems, emptiness searching for form on the formlessness of the cosmic white page.

The words somersaulted past my lips only once I redeemed the garbled texture of my right side from trauma's tirade. "Mind-Body Solutions," a virtual adaptive yoga community founded by Matthew Sanford, is my path back into fellowship and into my body. Before my spinal cord stroke, I never uttered the word "yoga," let alone engaged in its embodiment. But, as months tran-spire, I refine laughter, warrior pose, mountain pose, prayer pose, and camaraderie in silence, as I re-pose over and again, learning how to occupy space anew, redrafting my story as I witness my body's poise. I drape my shoulder blades downward and gently reach my sternum forward, a smile unfurling itself on the inside of my torso. I define home in my body, this remarkable assemblage of soft flesh that never left me and is now my tutor. Each member of "Mind-Body Solutions" congregation is a stanza, the physical geography between us being the necessary white of the page glowing with the ineffable. We carve positive and negative spaces, becoming something uniquely and unexpectedly united over Zoom.

We seek infinity within our disabled bodies. The oceans and continents between us seem to condense into a singularity. As we find ourselves in each other's eyes, undistracted by social media, we are beheld, heard, segmented—yet, somehow, transcendently whole. The delicate significance encrypted in our kinship of recognition, an almost hallowed well of self-reclamation, is so profound that it does not survive criticism or analysis. It demands plunging immersion in attentive presence. My bungled attempts to sift it through mental concepts only reduce its experiential nectar into a sort of scholarly chemical water diluted of its magic. We are not scared of our impermanence. We are coterminous with everything. We are all unbound. My right side is not my dark nemesis. Not anymore. I hug my unfeeling right shoulder with my left hand, returning my body to its nest, reestablishing my right riverbanks. I extend my compromised spinal cord from my sacrum to the crown of my head, gesturing with my right arm— my current third cousin, my soon-to-be neighbor, my will-be self. I will not begrudge you, no matter your recession from my brain.

I am an explorer rediscovering the unmapped and unmappable rugged terrain of my body. I am no longer afraid of the absences in my form, the lacunae in the logic that unwind and reincarnate us all in our incredible, untenable, and terrifying humanity. We are fragmented. We are undivided. We drink paradox. We are Armstrong on the moon of disability, showing the world how wondrous we are, how irreparably mortal we are. We know how to become our own constellations. There is a mixture of sorrow, divinity, and beauty that threads us through on the ledges of selves. We are evolving, alive multicolored watercolors that simultaneously cry and sing.

Part II
Pilgrimage

Epigraph

Continuity interrupted,
troubling my interaction with being.
 I am shocked out of time and space,
disoriented inside crisis.

Out of youth,
I'm in a different world—
apart, necessitating
renegotiating the narrative
over and again of
where I'm from,
how I survive being in my own
survival, how I revise
versions of subjectivity
that resist linearity.

I echo, echo
from the bind of
trauma.

Movement I
Reeling

Introduction

In this first section, separated into "movements" as if in a symphony, the speaker is first dealing with the reality of her new status as disabled. Here, she confronts her sorrow, a sensation that often threatens to engulf her. At interludes, she affirms her resolve, sustained by her parents' enduring commitment and by renewing her devotion to her creative practice. While the speaker is often frustrated with the limits of language, her sporadic writing develops into a devotional practice. She dives into herself and the new truth of her situation to uncover and awaken the components of the person that perished in the aftermath of her stroke, braiding her present with her past.

Synapse

a chasm between nerve fibers, a cleft of emptiness tinged
  with conversation,
silence boiling-over with feeling, molecular sign language,
back-and-forth shuttling of notes enveloped in
  membranes,
a billiards game between the closed fist of one neuron and
  the open webbed fingers of another,

a telegraph that wires us into now.

an invisible strip of highway,
a melting pot of migrating molecules
close to touching,
close to moving further away.

No one knows the expense of tomorrow, the price of the
    next moment.

two tributaries parting, an unfathomable juncture.

reunite me into the ionic flux of self.

I am falling out of synaptic connectivity with myself in my
    stroke's aftershocks-
insurmountable hacks in the firewall of the familiar.

I am refracted in this womb of silence, acutely acquainted
    with death and mortality,
churning in the infinite cosmos of suffering, my once
    incandescent passion
for synapses dropping away, a vicious amnesia of self—
the protruding experimenter enraptured in dialogue
    between pencil and laboratory notebook, the
    wedded learner of genetics, the mathematical zealot
    pouring over solutions spilling over reams of pages,
    the propulsive reader on a quest to excavate reasons
    coursing through fiction and fact, the lover of walks to
    nowhere with friends and abstract worlds of thought,
    that young woman on the brink of locating a first
    boyfriend—
a synapse not crossed,
now a synapse in still-motion,

a synapse uprooted, redacted
by a brainstem stroke.

The sky is falling today, opening up its broad navy arms to
   scatter
bits of white lace swirling into anonymity against
   pavement,
the celestial skinning its knees,
the heavens bleeding,
a synapse splitting overhead.

I am disoriented in this body I now share, a relentless
   ruthless rental, with disability.

Synapse me back into myself.

an assaulting break-up, flow in stagnation, hibernation of
   trauma, the bastille of my nervous system stormed.

I breed silence and am bred by it in this impregnable
   internal wintering.

All I can do is hold hands with my breath, my one lingering
   synapse from my before.

all else has decayed, a synapse shrugging, swallowing me
   whole.

Is 27 really the age of disappearance and demise?

I presumed it was the age of beginning—
the onset of innocence, the buoyant tide of emergence—
not an eruption of the synapse of self,
not vacuity of my honorably earned merit, grit and
   purpose.

Where did it all flee?

Is there a residence for the lost essentials of the soul in its
    infancy?

let me fall in love with synapses in their mechanistic
    majestic mystery again.

where have you gone, my once invincible ally—
my best friend of self, my brain,
my dear central nervous system, my bounty of life that
    locked me into being,
into becoming someone incalculably besotted by the
    universe.

world, synapse me back into marriage with you again.
Permit me to reside on shoulders of grassy mountains, to
    see into nature, to web myself into communion again
    with right half of my body derelict to my brain in this
    nightmare.

The world is still snapping its fingers without me.
But I hunger to harmonize with it, to feel it all again.

the meandering into and out of self, critical connectivity
    of consciousness, the unseen, unheard hum of the body
    yearning to tie
this world into a modicum of coherency.

And I will just be with this uncertain gash in my soul,
this incredulous synaptic division as I fall into disability's
    restraints,
into the arduous audacity to be with my body's
    adaptations,

because being mortal means carving out a synapse in the
   direction of mourning and surrender and another in the
   direction of hope and healing—
words whose definitions I have yet to meet but whose
   echoes I will
ricochet off interior lining until they synapse me into being
   anew beside you.

I implore you to absorb flashes of my wounds,
to metabolize mouthfuls or morsels of me,
to facilitate my slow coalescence into you,
your evolution through this space synapsing
onto pauses and poetics, networking us into belonging.

Discombobulated

This bleak present was shaded by palimpsests of my veered-from
past, by the irredeemable thrust of humanity, the discombobulating swell of sorrow and symphony. An untempered evocation
of naked disarray and dislocation churned, writhing syllables stirring commotion as they circle your tongue, the recurrent har-
assment of entropy unbound, the Big Bang quickening within
your should-have-been middle, the particles of your being interrupted, your unrecognizable limbs cast astray, hidden in the
dead of night ravenous for starlight—the once visceral urge to
be comprehensible and to comprehend, to unshackle ourselves
from our fragile bent towards discombobulation. A tinderbox of
mementos migrates up my esophagus, choking me in a landslide of disgruntled, disregarded memories of that other variety
of self—the severe incision of my stroke, the resection of my
becoming. Will the prisoners of war of our before bodies ever

return home? Oh, the plunge into my plundered form. I am mis-remembered by belief, by my aghast nervous system ghosted by its reflection. I deflect. I refract. I refrain from this discombobulating instant. This one block of text hungry for pause welcomes no relief, no exit, ensnaring you in this snaking trauma as it vines its way into me, making words out of itself so I become we. I throb to no longer sanction the could-have-beens that break you more than you are already broken. This call and response between me and myself gives way to disharmony. The cognitive dissonance of this stroke unmakes my brain, unprescribes me of the necessity to know. Experience has cornered us. Time misbehaves; it skips, stutters, grinds to a halt, forgets us as we forget ourselves. Someone, bless us as we fall through loopholes in the connective tissue of our lives. I am a pariah. I am floodgates juddering open. I am disintegrating cells, decomposing rational, a peeling away of fantastic illusions. Scream with me until we are caught by exhaustion, drugged into a stupor of our own tears. My uncoordinated legs no longer cooperate but bully me into abnegation, a total subtraction of my psyche. We are bird nests lurching out of barbed branches. We are lost in the clogged artery of humanity. Shards of our souls careen out of us. Have you been sidelined too? We are pruned pulses under tension, under turmoil. We are left bereft. We are closed doors. We are petrified wood. The loathing scorching our bloodstreams forces us to sit with the hours, leakage of time, wounds that may never scab over. I desire to let go of my life story, pick up this new thread the cosmos is tossing my way. I am teetering on the cusp of sorrow, hanging onto the brink of suffering, legs dangling off the cliff of trauma and paralyzing fear, eyes wide shut against the mayhem of my cracked visual field. I am respiring and holding my breath, gliding through the panic of existence as I gaze into the tailspin of a panic attack. Despite the passage of a year—during which sensation has not inked its way back into my right side, during which all that has been lost has not been retrieved—my jaw quivers in fear, gripping me tightly into chokehold of trepidation of the known, rather than of the unknown. I perspire at the material life has made of me, not at the future that has been abducted from within, not at the loss of hearing in my right ear, not at the deletion of my system's once innate, mellifluous homeostatic rhythm, but at what I expect—the symptoms that leave me spinning, reaching through the dark for an object to steady me, on an invisible roller coaster drenched in frozen solitude. How do you cope with the paradoxes that ripple through your life? Let us learn to be with them together. This universe is half-remembered. I still look at my unfeeling right side as though I were looking into the eyes of the intimate exotic, desperately resolved to trace a prior link, a partial bridge, a tattered synapse. I have become an observer of the world, an avalanche of an organism dwelling on the other side of wherever I once was, an outcast, a perplexed victim of circumstance. I am stuck in liminality, in the bewildering middle ground between here and there, between being and not being, between everything and nothing. I will hold onto this moment. I will hold onto this breath. I hold onto the grueling frustration to be. I will invite these unwelcome guests into my being. The monsoon of mankind nearly swallows me; I am unhinged, dismembered, gasping on the precipice of desolate despair. We are the problem. We are the prescription. We are the pill. We are the placebo. The massive weight of the words we spiral into being, out of being, around the artistry of being, might be all we have. We have been bleached out, weathered to burnt crips. We are terrible, vulnerable, invaluable, textured into textiles of trauma. There is something in me still kicking. Can you feel it? Can you hear it? Please wage this war with me on the frontier of my stroke. I do not need to squeeze the prior and current species of my being into the same breath—both are here, undeniable. Sometimes, church bells do not ring through the pain, but the agony is stark razor-sharp agony, without the varnish of song. We yell, keep ourselves at bay, squirm and squint to see our footpath back into the shoes that once clattered against boulevards in dance to reverberating why-nots, the smiles uncoiling through our expressions with dexterous irrationality. We live in multiple directions, photons swinging on the discombobulated atmosphere of the multiverse. I yearn for this strangled blow of misery to no longer be my chorus line. I am playing a new rhythm, asserting a portion of myself never before realized. Come into my phalanx as we rail against the blur of disability.

We fall short of summation

I am the cost of what nobody can undo.

I am not stronger for my survival against steep medical
    odds.
I am transformed, the crucible, but irreversibly weakened
beneath the mallet of the debt
of that beyond the white-picket fence
of everything I can never control.

There is no half-life to this tragedy.

It simply languishes and lambasts alongside me for the
  duration—
sometimes skating beside a sliver
of hope oftentimes serrated with rage,
a throttling pendulum that craters through my tenses as
I clamber my way through these
graceful and graceless uncertainties.

This is the in-between where no language sinks its toes,
where steadiness does not localize home.

Show me how to walk through
this world without smacking my shins against touchstones
  of trauma.

I once found sublime solace
in what I presumed to be natural symmetry—
in fractals manifest in that pinecone,
in the continuous flux between day and night.
I saw mathematics beneath the transparent veil of
  nature—
an undercurrent of steel truth running like a cosmic
  unstoppable wire,
igniting everything into almost Christmas.

I never thought it could be otherwise.

I took this decadent view of the world and ran with it,
as though it were divine veracity,
as though life itself were a kite buffering wind I could steer
  in accordance
with my inner compass—
that magnet that magnetized me to

the wonders of the world once so plentiful.

You could call me naïve.

You could call me buoyantly optimistic.

You could call me deliciously at ease.
But that is no longer me.

My worldview shattered into a charade
in synchrony with my trauma that breaks me anew each
     morning.

Mathematics metamorphosed into the dust of discipline,
something separate from nature,
which I have learned lacks symmetry, is maliciously,
     radically
and radioactively asymmetric—
a game of chance, an uprooting roll of the dice
deprived of anything the world will teach you about logic,
about Dostoyevsky's *Crime and Punishment*.

Localize the crime preceding my unending current of
     punitive measures
waterboarding me in a pool of suffering,
depths deepening by the day, the hour.

I am losing faith in the world, in myself,
in what it means to endure
in a body that no longer remembers how to function.

At age 27, I am at a loss for everything—
too debilitated
to use the restroom on my own,
to walk,

to sense anything
on the right side of my being.

I no longer remember
hunger, thirst, the beauty of
bilateral symmetry incarnate.

I miss the mathematics once ingrained in my own body,
in my perspective, however fallacious.

I wish I could exchange
those falsehoods for this unbridled brutal truth.

I do not need this type of knowing gnawing at the rough
  exterior
of my soul, splintering everything
I once thought I knew into specs of despondency.

There must be more to life than this heap of hardship—
this mass whose load accumulates with time.

I am trying to carry it all.
Can you bear some of the burden with me?

But I fear that the
integral of my sorrow and suffering
is decomposing me beyond repair.

I am not looking to overcome anything.

I am not looking for rebirth.

Are you?

All I yearn for now is a trickle of repose—
a sun-shower of light to descend upon the darkness, to
  become mildly better than I am.

I do not think the world can give me more, so I am scared
   to long for more,
to be let down by feckless and careless reality.

My skin is thickening by the day, so I need the light
to come quickly before all of my pores
permanently close, refuse to let it in.

You are the story you spirograph out of what life does to
   you.

So let us climb out of the woodwork of disability into the
shafts of light illuminating the darkest dark,
igniting the matchsticks of our beings
as we hatch our way into becoming,
despite the mop of despair raking through the mind.

Torrent of grief

It is impossible to truly quantify loss, to approach its asymptote, to gently knock it on the shoulder and say this is it, this is me, these are my circumstances and my situation. No one can come to terms with the utter devastation, the demolition, the ruin of its toll on the psyche, the life, the mind, the spirit, the body, which spills out in all directions, a carton of milk impetuously thrown on the floor, seeping into nooks and crannies on kitchen tiles. When it hits you, slaps you across the cheek, it overruns you, full steam ahead, without conscious consideration, without apologies, without warning. Suddenly, you are ambushed in the crossfire and crossed wires, bemused by what has become your life—upended by the distortions that capsize the foundation of person you presumed you were. In a millisecond, decades are stripped away. Time curtly unspools, unravels itself, undoes you. And just when the loss seems like it is at a loss, like it can hold no more loss, like it is oozing beyond its own container and you are over it, it hits you again but at a different angle, punching you, its knuckles bloody, in the stomach, leaving you hugging your knees into your chest on the floor, feeling it as though it were the first time it struck you. I was 27, feet stationed on the launchpad of becoming. I was ready for almost anything, or so I miscalculated.

But then this haphazard stroke, the precursor to agony, came down like a hailstorm that never quits. What resides now aside from this breath in this body, aside from this sentence coming out of these lips, emerging into coherency out of nothing? Because our circumstances are, at the end of the day, unfortunately for me, more defining than our genes and nothing, save the narrative we parse out of impoverished marginality, can override them. There is no signal, no control panel, no reset button that can turn the dial backwards or sideways on your reality so that you know: you are not your vestibular symptoms, you are not your lack of depth perception, you are not your incontinence, you are not your ability to hear out of only one side of your head, you are not your loss of vision in your right eye, you are not the burning pain that lingers from the bleed inside your brain. But you are. You know you are. There are times, and there are days, and there are moments when the grief sneaks up on you like a child playing who gently taps you on the shoulder, ready to come out of the closet in which you have not yet checked, ready to knock you down, to make you fall on the ground and cry tears that have no end, middle, or beginning, but simply roll out of you, a decimating current of waves rolling through the ocean. I may always be like this. I may always never feel the right side of my body. I am petrified of this very sentence. I am petrified of this very breath. I know that I should be grateful for simply being alive—for being able to breathe, despite my compromised brainstem, the epicenter of so many vital functions.

But most days, blessings are not what I feel. I feel cursed. I feel grief. I feel victimized. I feel shorn of an identity I dedicated so many decades to build as a student, as a scientist, as a writer, as a painter, as a walker, as a bipedal human who loved adventuring through the world without an agenda.

There are reasons to keep fighting, to keep wishing for a better tomorrow. And yet, there are reasons tantamount in quantity to give in, to relent, to say enough is enough, to cry, and to not know when the cry is over, to feel like I am irreconcilably lost, distressingly neglected, helplessly misunderstood, impossibly bypassed, despairingly overlooked, massively downtrodden by life and entropy, the brittle circumstances that now chain me.

But I have learned to say several things to myself each day that convince me to cultivate hope, to embody courage.

I am more of a paradox than a problem.

I possess more fight than relent.

I am more of an advocate for myself than a hapless victim.

But some moments feel much safer than others. Some moments make me want to scream, to slice off the right side of my body. I miss you, right side. I miss sensing you, knowing you, letting you define me. There is a plethora of loss buried under tragic pain.

There is ample grief emulsified with hope. The two go together, twin sisters, but they never venture alone.

I am trying to delineate what a life can mean inside of a body as fractured, as debilitated as my own. The fight is draining me, and I am being drained from it, feeling as though I am being hoisted up shard by shard out of a deep cranny in the Earth as my will weakens. I never speak the echoing question of should I pursue this moment, the thought that taunts and haunts, the penetrating interrogation, the unsayable syllables that unlatch a torrent of grief, abducting me of all that endures. Let us blister, bluster, bruise, blush, and bloom out of the thoughts that trample us more than our traumas.

Concussed pronouns

Through the portal of words—
a frame around the portrait of existence impervious to
    language,
I awaken into the passenger seat within this disabled
    body—
this haunted, hallowed or hollow
glass vessel chemically broken down into constituent parts
I once thought were forever locked into bondage as
I decomposed molecular structures
I supposed solely sat within the neat-penciled purview of
    chemistry classrooms.

Where is Elly?

Where is Elly's purpose that clung to her skin like freckles?

I refrain into the abyss of self.

She is a library book eternally on lease lingering on
the shelves of the universe—
out of step with herself,
out of vogue,
shaken up,
buried alive—
her potential enshrined, clandestine
between her soul and Earth.

She, like the dwellers in Plato's cave, mistook the shadows
   of the world
for reality until she morphed into her shadow—
was flipped inside out, and the unreal bones of the
world became transparent,
too bright and visible,
a biting light she often has to shut her eyes against.

Now, her unanswerable questions wear ankle weights.

The world is no longer a looming textbook to devour.

She watches her resolve
slip and nearly fall a thousand times.

My mind blows a fuse at what has become of me,
at my past participle I now call her,
more a distant relative than a rendering of self.

These words are my way out, or my way in—
they gnaw and rake, a hunger pooling in the pit of my
   stomach.
I crave to read my way
into this incarnation of self not fully realized.

I am wasting away, not from hunger or thirst,

but from something spiritual that words can dance
around but never fully penetrate—
from the smile that once inched its way towards the
    corners of my eyes,
careening me into a parachute of being,
a dancing dazzling creature
carving out a nexus in the world—
a devoted reader of all words, a singer in the rain,
a soul entangled in a body that relished experiences that
    have
indiscriminately evaporated into the no longer feasible
in the after of traumatic upheaval that corseted me in the
    bolted room of disability.

My stroke relegated me to a watcher of nature through my
    windowpane,
leading me to wonder when my bleak winter will yield to
    spring—
when my breaking will be broken so the cycle that
spins the Earth will kick into the core of my being,
when I will be a part of things instead of
apart from things.

And, in my own physical decomposition,
certain segments of mind never before realized clicked
    into unity.
I begin to contemplate animals and what their
dreams feel like without language and conscious thought,
if their sense of awe outstrips our own,
what this entity we call time—
the one residue of reality I cannot seem to misplace no
    matter my effort—

truly is, if it is, when I am out of place,
within its unflinching grip,
what becomes of our past exposures and experiences,
if the soul sleeps with the body or if its eyes reside wide-
    open nocturnally.

And, despite the plight of mind,
the body possesses a coping ritual of its own,
a magical connection occurring when I assume mountain
    pose—
grounding my sit bones,
extending through the crown of my head,
and delicately inching my shoulder blades towards each
    other—
steering my way against the tides of loss
that shrink me into
the despair that crushes my heart a million times a day
into someone who is gradually learning
how to expand in all directions,
reaching through the dark for the possible, even though I
    know the
right side of my being—
the half of me leeched
of sensation since my stroke—
is my Roman coliseum, my crumbling walls of Jericho,
my erosive yet alive part of my becoming
I must adopt into the pillar of a rewritten self
if I aim to live beyond the confined
tangled vines of trauma and start again
from the subatomic particles
of being incurably human.

Prayers through ruins

At 28, I dwelt in the rubble
of my beset central nervous system.

I am unlearning my innate impulsivity—
my hunger to hurry everywhere and nowhere,
foot slamming the accelerator
ornamenting my résumé
with academic accolades,
through boyfriends and other firsts,
to thicken the substance being into experiential agar.

But now, I am ghoulishly pared back,
stumbling through the wreckage of trauma,
learning life fails to comply with logic,
with any seasoning
of intelligence
we douse.

I am learning patience—
how to linger in empty pockets of time,
how to do nothing save
for the massive undertaking
of attending to everything
that already is,
how to hunker down,
to RSVP to nature's invitation
to dwell in the exquisite minutia
of this unscripted moment.

Even in this sick room,
I inhale something divine,

cosmically essential particles,
as I listen to rain tickling a dance on windowpanes.

My void of sensation on the right side of
my spinal cord distorts the text of my flesh
into novel with all of the pages
on the right side excerpted
so the story inescapably
reads nonsensically—
an accidental rendition of
Lewis Carroll's "Jabberwocky."

Natural landscape is often
frustratingly inaccessible.

But I am not despondent, as I know I am engaging
in the same task as that tree over there,
as that fly pecking at the sill.

We are all gathering celestial atmosphere into our
    bodies—
be they broken or not yet broken—
siphoning out oxygen to sublimely nurture ourselves,
to assemble the magnificently transient out of identical
    raw material.

Unlike the roots nestled beneath the soil,
the caterpillar perched on that branch,
I contain multitudes
of fear, sadness, a sense of my own ending, my own
    mortality.

I contemplate God—
what that word, so loaded by our world with judgment,

dogma, didactics
and scriptural strictures, actually is.

I wonder, as I attempt and fail over and again
to educate my brain to walk on a leg it no longer feels,
as nauseating pain darts down my left back and leg—
my only leg my nervous system has yet to reject—
if the grasses or the trees ever bluster about divinity.

Swiftly, birdsong rings through my pain.

Trees, clouds, the ceiling over it all,
cannot help but
sing.

The tortured voice in my head grows quiet.

I am unfastened from the stronghold of trauma,
its unpayable taxes on body and soul.

If that melody dangling in the sky
is not a prayer,
tell me what is.

Residue

I binge on scanty resources at my disposal.
Empty of hunger and thirst, I am satiated with indolence,
solitude, darkness, drenching despair—
eatables that lambast, accost me within sharp elbows of
  disability.

emotion curdles through my fractured form, a waltz of
  silent surrender.

I am forgotten.

I am immobilized.

a dancer no longer.

What are these feet for if not to slide across floorboards to
  melodic riffs?

dreams emigrate into waking, obscuring the profound
  brutality of
this phantasm of presence, this self-erasure leaving but
  residual outskirts of my penciled before.

I miss you, my prior variant of being,
my once belonging,
my life minus this brainstem stroke.

How did this happen at age 27?

existence refuses to comply with human arithmetic—
we live lives forward and backward, within the grand
  delusion of linearity,
but do not have access to rewind time.

I throb to reside once again in untempered integrals and
  derivatives.
Return me to the residue of that redacted document of
  being.

I am stark, naked.

please find me beneath these palimpsests.

Are you there?

I drink and eat, succumbing to my own hibernation.

my sheared synapse washed away demands of the
   stepwise function of being.
How I thrived within the embrace of my previous draft.

now, I am but attentive to myself, treading uncensored
   thoughts.

This world a world away.

The pen of my vocal cords jogs to keep pace with my
   observant eyes.
Oh, this brain—
dismantled, casted, dependent but ineffably,
undeniably present.
this is my scrawl on the bark of the cosmos.

Here I am.

I will locate my residues of self, so I can once again emerge
   in inky black,
assimilate to more than but a residue.

A fountain in the desert

I will never crack the case of this fugue state of
heightened presence,
a poetic enmeshing in the net of the world,
a lost finding of the self beyond the girl of my before.

These ever-deepening waters are almost painful,
excessively meaningful, aching for a reverse intervention,
for a flood of all of the drugs in all of the pharmacies of
   mankind.

I will never catch up with the causal thread

that sunk me wide-eyed into this dark underworld.

I am drifting through the desert,
the desolate and despondent red land harsh beneath my
    feet
as they tread with neither path nor destination.

For whom on this Earth truly knows where they are going?

Is there really a path paved by anyone, save for cosmic
    design?

Call it God.

Call it fortune.

Call it by whatever name you desire.

Labels only constrict the labeler.

Do not barricade more cages for yourself.

We are all atoms loosely
sutured together into skin and bones,
into outrageous laughter,
dismaying tears, our bodies bruised or broken,
yet capable of untangling
themselves into something ravishingly raw,
something magnificently mortal.

Here but a moment.

There is no cure for the human condition—
no prescription to fill at the pharmacy
to remedy the tickle in your throat that causes you to
    choke on thoughts of your
own transience—

your petrifying and pulchritudinous
knowledge of death, intelligence you shun at every turn.

Do not run away frantically from this word.

It only hurts you.

It is only language.

There is but this one life you have, this one opportunity to
chisel a dazzling crystal of meaning out of the soul
  flapping within.

Your wings, like mine, may be clipped,
may be inept to fly, may be fraught by whatever
  immobilizes.

But there is a nugget of gold
buried within your recesses.

So take a shovel to dig in internal soil,
so that you may know
you can become something susceptible to sparkling,
no matter how feeble and ashen you feel.

And the birds are soaring
overhead as the world careens, as humans decompose,
as we become,
as we begin.

The sun still rises each morning.

Each day calls your name to attention.

Each moment is the silent alarm
you refuse to hear sounding within your heart,
informing you that it is brand new, that you can ordain

yourself into novelty, that you can integrate your pieces,
no matter how scattered and segmented
they may feel within the parchment of your skin.

You are still here.

Bear witness to what is.

Sit within the infinite arms of your pain and sadness,
and let them tell you their story so you may come to know
   yourself.

Prepare for flight, but do not flee.

You are only running away from your truest self—
a respiring being on the fulcrum of
chance circumstance,
a miraculous happenstance that
happens to be right here.

Let everything that is just settle.

As long as you still are,
you can still become.

Where can I find you?

This body is at once a miraculous survivor,
a definitive resistor of medical statistics,
and a vessel of profoundly inarticulable despair inflamed
   with
blasts of pain demanding to be felt,
abbreviating attention into near oblivion.

This fortress of cells from which she

magically emerges is supersaturated with undigestible
  trauma—
fraught fibers of the spirit languish unprocessed.

How can she come to terms, to a reckoning,
with this body, with this disability,
so disparate from the life blockaded in her before?

There was a girl whose smile was a lightning bolt—
an engine stockpiled with kinetic energy; innocence
  unencumbered.

There was a girl on the corner of womanhood, on a brink
  of firsts-
an initial trail of boyfriends,
a trailblazing career,
an assortment of peers,
an apartment of her own,
a garden she would have grown thrusting with
organically wild beauty, kept unkempt nature.

But this girl is but a dream,
and her dreams but ash scattered through my soul,
through every cell coursing through me,
a medley of division and retraction.

She now contends with the unimaginable in the after of
  her stroke,
her erasure from her once lush existence.

She now references herself primarily in the third person,
often incapable of coping with the ruthless reality
that she is me, that her life is mine.

Part of her aches to be met by
a force other than defeat,
to grow bigger in space,
to expand her boundaries,
to shirk,
or at least to shrink,
fear of her own emptiness.
Her body is not afraid of loneliness,
but her mind is.

She forfeits her newfound strength
over and again,
an Alzheimer's of soul.

Her dilapidated body
creeks with life.

It is only her mind that is crestfallen.
It is only her mind that causes her spine
to cavern concave at exile, because
this feels like her only recourse—
prayer inverted.

It is only her mind that needs the words
to speak insignificance into being.

Her body delivers her back to life.

Her mind, not her body, feels the disempowerment of her
    trauma.

She needs to acclimate to
the quiet that infiltrated the right half
of her body.

She is still breathing.

But there is no end to her sorrow, a snake encircling her
   calf,
intractably weighing her down, inertia unsettling her,
stagnantly stationing her in a bottomless abyss flowing
   with darkness.

But an epiphany dawns on her, as she stares at the
   darkness out of her left eye
that even the blackest, most disconsolate
shade of night is freckled with specks of light,
perhaps the only eternal living thing on this planet.

The light is everything.

Time is but a construct.

Forever is an idea she wraps her tongue
around over and again.

She likes its taste, the flavor of tenses winding around each
   other,
the past melding with the present.

She craves to enlist empowerment to trek
through quicksand pulling her
under at an accelerating clip from the darkness
to all the light within her and beyond her.

She wants to open her eyes—
both the one that is
visually intact and the one that
sees the world as though it were an impressionist
   painting—

to let all the light in till she's illuminated,
a glowing creature, however broken,
so that she can begin to relate to herself
in the first person again,
so that she cultivates hints of light into the ally,
into the laughter, the buoyancy she once called her own.

She hungers to find a footpath home,
whatever that word has come to mean.

But more than anything,
she yearns to live before she must
surrender her bones to the Earth that made her.

The waste land

T S. Eliot's magnum opus, a tangled tumbling dissonance
   of zeitgeist
swimming in a distraught desert of literary allusions—
a "heap of broken images,"
"fear in a handful of dust,"
an ocean of "fragments I have shored against my ruins."

I am finally ready to swivel my head to the rear-view of my
   mind,
to rummage through my *Waste Land*,
to prune layers of fossils:
a reservoir of still-lives
sluicing, churning, undulating with dynamic bitter
   nostalgia,
seasickness of the psyche,
the past linking arms with presence, a gesture of queer
   intimacy at first encounter.

Time falls into disrepute,
out of its socket.

Quanta of light ignite the flickering lantern in my soul,
exposing all I have buried as these decibels
crash against my tongue.

thermodynamics capsizes all—
even "dead men have lost their bones,""rock" is "without
   water,"
Eliot's sole seer a blind prophet.

Truth emerges at moments punctuated by breakage—
a point of access occluding a slipping into mundane
   rituals,
when you are prohibited from asking
"What shall we do today? What shall we ever do?"

You see the rigidity of routine as though it were a
viewed from a great distance,
a blurring whoosh of color,
when you are locked out of your future *Waste Land*.

against my will, I am more of an anthropologist than active
   participant in life,
the chasm developing between me and
my once inhabited *Waste Land*—
a forced planetary migration,
a closing of the gates as trauma leaves me alone
with myself, my *Waste Land* resounding
against the weary floorboards of my mind.

show me serenity and freedom inside this disabled cage.

I need this instant to be less razor sharp, less bountiful of
    the sacred.

I yearn to return to *The Waste Land* in real, not in recalled,
    time.

I no longer fear the sieve of my brain,
the separation exacted between me and becoming.

I pray I am not too late to commence.

Is forgetting happening right now?

I knock furtively, my first dim and weary, against the old
    door of twisted memory,
blowing through thick layers of grime cloaking the surface
    of past shadows,
switching on the lantern in my soul.

I will tell myself her story until its echo envelops me,
leaves an etching, a residue, a footfall.

I want to save her.

I want to set her free.

She is me, I whisper to myself,
trembling awe drenched in trepidation.

do not let me remember.

Do not let me forget.

These letters leap into silence, into each other, with
    urgency, fueled with kinetic energy between me and the
    page, between the page and your gaze.

I conjure myself.

How quickly it all vanishes, diaphanous steam merging
  into atmosphere.

We disintegrate into nothing, into silence.

through the windowpane of reverie, I cozy up to tufts of
  curls
roaming through dandelions, to the studious student
  surging on the waves of Latin
binomial nomenclature, scientific theorems, Fermat's
  enigma,
vines of memorized numbers compressed into pi
that once lulled me into blissfully logical slumber.

my injury abducted my right side—
a zoo of body parts that convulse of their own accord.
I'm in time's purgatory.

Alien to myself in a splinter of a shivering
moment, its mouth still ajar two years after death nearly
  found me at age 27.

the world does not offer the bounty of two weeks' notice
  before we expire,
atoms mulling over estrangement.

Part of me still moves jauntily through stacks in Widener
  Library—
locating interior audits in Euler and Darwin, in Shakespeare
  and Eliot,
finding myself until I slid out of academia,
rerouted, strokes tore me asunder, stapled me into furious
  fear.

I am not where I'm supposed to be.

Are you?
Is anyone?

in my bleary-eyed, nightmare vision,
I am glimpsed,
gone.

I take a single oblique, obliterating look as I trespass within.

I amble through the dark inferno of dreams toppled, a
    forest so overgrown with rupture.

She is still visiting Newton's laws, quantifying quantum
    physics,
stooped over evolutionary genetics texts, crafting scientific
    papers,
combing through articles, parsing Tolstoy and
    Dostoyevsky, typing frantically as though she knew she
    bled time before the universe roared its deafening truth
into my ears, dispatching all causal knots assiduously
    roped together.

I am her.
She is me.

we are both there and here,
nowhere and somewhere,
untraceable, choreography of sun and clouds.

I search for hope so I can catch it,
a bug beneath a cup,
let its pulse quicken in me so my *Waste Land*
becomes less ruination, more a rainforest,

so I no longer scare myself, slices of me entombed,
specimens preserved in the mousetrap of memory, so I
   can
thread the needle of being into a quilt that confers
   comfort, tranquility.
Because we are all lost, are all longing to find our way with
   only time
and the blindness that comes with loss to upend us
and then, suddenly, to help us mend our way home.

Grow in darkness

Suffering is my vocation, my trump card,
the merciless expertise the universe
foisted upon me to grow into,
to grow out of,
to grow despite.

There were ebullient words,
surfeit syllables floating mellifluously through fingertips—
the typist equivalent of a concert pianist,
I composed my route into existence,
inking meaning out of uncertainty,
a mainstay of my bittersweet becoming.

There was once a profusion of expression—
so much diction,
so many explanations,
so much understanding in the ears of others
despite the barren display
of my connective tissue disease—
a scarce invisible economy of braces—

nothing anyone could point to decipher my ailment.

But there were sentences,
definitions, fellowship—
cohort bruised by congruent elements,
a sticky sense that I was unalone, if not curable.

But now, six months into the bloodstained white knuckles
   of
emergency—
even more so than my
spontaneous cerebrospinal fluid leaks,
my hydrocephalus,
my cervical instability—
the words ploddingly turn,
amble my way,
not through cadence of keystrokes,
but through lips,
hesitatingly flowing across my synapses
at jerky unaccustomed velocity
but with intention they always gathered:
to unify me,
to make me whole where it counts.

However, in the face of this prosaic comeback,
I am an indefinite article
in this redacted document.

No number of interwoven syllables can reach
the unnerving,
paralyzing, perplexing, devouring.

No letters match the boiling-over
of not feeling,

of waking and groping with my left hand for my right,
crestfallen that my brain is ransacked, hacked.

Where is that girl I used to be?
Where are her passions, hobbies, drive to dive into
   everything?

I search for the fearless creature, but feel as though I am
   slaving to
capture water with a fishing net—
pores too monstrous to retrieve that which I crave.

Where is that girl who carved time as an artist chisels
   marble?

I miss the brainstem I never before contemplated.
I miss the sensation I never before thought about sensing.
I miss the easy gait that once flew into my feet innately
   with sunrise.
I miss the organism I once inhabited.

My past no longer feels like mine.

The present is so beleaguering, so exhaustively taxing, so
   unnervingly terrifying.

The future is out of bounds, a tongue lost.

There is no foreshadowing what lies ahead when you are
   your
own prelude in a minor key—
the lone survivor of your species.

If only I could novelize, clock out of, this crisis.

What about the absence of prescience?

What about my parents?

Their astounding commitment to consistency,
to my survival of this incursion,
their will to extract and extrapolate their girl—
whited out, her iridescent past blowing in
whimpering winds of yesterday,
now but a palimpsest,
an ellipsis trailing off
without her.

I am unfixable,
chewed up by the incident
that incited my error.

Swaddle me, words.

My father yet aims to ward off danger, to promulgate a
    defensive strategy.

He hunts for an oracle.

We all zigzag through sea-changes at divergent rates.
But a furtive underbelly unique to this horrific situation
    stills me.

There is growth in this dark nexus to begin again,
but no return to factory settings.

There is an eerie and shocking blank canvas
waiting for me to watercolor—
a motley of primary colors and tears—
who I want to program into a self as I
subtract what I can excavate from my past.

Even if this project of being occupies years,

I will endure the labor throbs
within the womb of trauma as I sharpen my essence anew.

Unlearning

The sensory world once called my name through a mega-phone, issuing forth laundry lists of potentials blurred into the atmosphere. Now, fenced into myself, my name is but a whisper through spaces in barbs—a sound I strain to hear. Feelings bri-dled through me on horseback now meander hesitantly on inau-dible tiptoes, falter to walk at all, in cavities in my right side. I am washing out. I recall slotting being into boxes of thoughts piled, an impenetrable fortress of intelligence coming out of experi-ence. There is no storage for life inside conceptual construction, no hard drive for meaning within words we compress into stories we tell ourselves. At its core, life is fundamentally incommunica-ble. You cannot catch me in language because I cannot catch myself. The world is already so full. There is no need to suffuse it with meaning. I am learning to let go of the interpretive structure of the universe, to permit the world reveal itself before me, in all of its tumultuous and tremulous immediacy. Life is ungraspable. I am liberated from the shackles of needing to explain myself to you, to myself. There is needling freedom in my divestiture. There is liberation in letting go, even if the sensations that arise are absences, deprivations, and deficiencies. I unlearn. I don't fear death. Let's sweat out every petrifying thought together. At this point, after glaring at it in the eye for over 13 months, I am not even sure what fear is—the run-on conversation between us stretching into outrageous obscenity—what anything is other than what acutely occurs now, here. I will let it all settle unsettled, despite the rattling of my spirit against these tolls. I use language, but I refuse to let language use me, to weave me in the loom of human classifications that will never justify all. I will never have the words to offload myself. Here I am. This is now. Let it be.

Ensnared in ember

That girl who danced through wild grass, dangled on the
    ledge of sprouting wings
and soaring skyward, plucked dandelions from Earth
and blew with gentle might unencumbered,
shedding potential in concentric circles around her
    becoming—
nature's invisible embrace, a symbiosis of soul and seed,
silent effervescent conversation met with giggles and
    wonder
at the preferable preverbal encounter between
    untarnished innocence and emergence—
now leached of vitality, the frame frozen, belonging
beside entomological artifacts on museum shelves,
disposed by the world that was once at her disposal.

The puzzles of her youth now find their way into the
    epicenter of
her composition, decomposing and recomposing her
over and again, as ribs dislocate on the right side of her
    being
derelict by her brain, that organ once capable of
reducing complex matrices into transparent sense,
that element subsumed and subjugated it all—
mellifluous tangle of neurons she presumed her compass,
her gravity, her birthright,

her mode of absorption,
transforming everything into sweets she could consume
   to satiate her appetite for
facts fencing in the known world she deduced to be the
   sum of the universe,
like the cosmos could be siphoned into one grand
   equation
topped-off with a multitude of variables
she could gradually resolve over the spell of her one
   lifetime.

This thought once steadied her, once captivated reality
   someplace
between her palm and a calculator.

Oh, what a gift:
the delusion of naïve certainty.

Give it back to me, world, if only for a moment.

But now, she distances herself
from herself,
has opened up a network of pathways in that same brain
   that lead her to herself
from behind the smokescreen of pronouns at a remove—
an internal smog that is at once
an escape valve and a hiding place, a halfway house—
within her very essence.

She deeply misses the lens of intelligence, logic born of
   unadulterated being.

She only wanted to begin her life,
or perhaps to reach its middle distance,

to bisect reality, but never thought her way across the
   finish line.

Does anyone truly cross such a line in this one lifetime?

But now, I am bemused about
my blurred boundaries, about my own pronouns,
about whether I can bear these unbearable sharp teeth.

I attempt to accept the right side of my body
I can no longer feel nor control, to renegotiate my contract
   with gravity,
to move gracefully in a body that feels more like a
   penitentiary,
more like a dark shadowy landscape mourning light.

I am overwrought by loss,
by the exasperating and excruciating heaviness of my right
   side—
two entire skyscrapers reeling from my torso whose pivot-
   points I know not.

This massive absent presence winnows me down to what I
   cannot live without—
the irony of outrageous laughter through tears,
volumes of stories I thrust my way into,
music of silence and euphonious chords,
a jumble of blank pages for me to fill and, most of all,
my mother's eyes staring back at me,
witness to my suffering, saying something unsayable—
sandpaper smoothing out the harsh edges of my soul
splintering into bits of self-scattering though the breeze,
the universe now ironically plucking and blowing out my
   internal dandelions,

so I must muster costly courage to renovate my entire life,
to become the architect and interior decorator of a self I
  have yet to face.

Empathy that completes me

What is this undefinable article we call home?

Is it the whistle of wind shuttering through oak branches?
Is it the taste of Tennessee grits seeped in butter?

Is it the touch of your mother's palm clenching your left
  shoulder?

Is it the emptiness of being generated by easy breath in
  silence—
a sabbath of offloading,
a letting go of all of the threads,
distending your perspective into a capacious opening?

Is it a glance at a mountain erect and firmly rooted?

Or is it the converse—being unmoored
from your empirical formula of existence without
succumbing to the urgency to quit
the unstoppable and unspeakable enduring?

Perhaps it is letting the darkness envelope you, a sheet
  gliding without friction.

Perhaps it is right here, in the spellbinding infinity of
  attentive presence.

Perhaps it is a sense of safety, even if that feeling is long
  gone,

as fleeting as a thought in an amnesiac's mind.

Perhaps home is housed in fossils of memory,
even when you feel like compounding disinterest of loss
thresholds crossed.

Perhaps home is located within the crosshairs of tragedy
    exactly
when your mother embraces your entire being—
uniting the side of your spinal cord,
on which sensation and awareness have fled,
and the other side on which feeling is a lightbulb, always
    on,
imparting you with an acute degree of completion in your
    physical disrepair,
touch's edgeless voice telling you that you are enough,
that life will make you into something challengingly
    different,
but into something nonetheless
out the abiding fragments of your spirit.

And out of my mother's compassion,
I itch to reflect affection lubricating her blues,
to eschew the pretense of pretend,
to paint myself in real, unmitigated color.

Home is the life I have—
the horrific, the magnificent—
the not coming to terms with this world
I astonish myself for continuing
to embrace
in spite of everything,
because of everything.

Parallax

the shift you note in the world by shifting your seat within,
practicing musical chairs without music.

Meaning soaking through the soil, saturating the soul with
a paucity of language, resides in the province of the
  eyes—
in parallax—
not in the astounding anatomical outward gaze,
but in the seeing in,
in implicating us in our own
unique perspectival knitting between
the world we have subsumed beneath the headline of
reality and our own interiority.

Meaning was not created in step with our corporeality.

We are the forerunners to parallax—
inner doors we neglect that open to
fields blooming with purpose.

Perhaps we fear what we may find within ourselves,
so we search for something the universe
never tilled on our behalf beyond our vulnerability.

The invocation to inquire within,
the willingness to meet
our own quiet tragedies.

But it is precisely because of our
unshakable intimacy with death, our acceptance of
Camus' invitation to "live to the point of tears"—
simultaneously befriending loss and marveling at

this exquisite unfolding—
the shape of the wooden toothbrush,
the circular rim of the paper cup,
the metronomic rhythm of the heart,
the piercing throb of pain—
too readily skipped over,
the mind tempted to template the future rather than lean
  into the now.

The beautiful sadness that the nuances of
truths snaking theses
scrawny verses are always
paths diverging
between
me
and you.

The fact that a flood of language will never do justice to
  the
internal silence swimming with memory,
to Eckhart's "uncreated aspect of the soul"—
this secluded essence of self
that is ours to mold if
we courageously confront the
daunting irrefutable reality
that we must give
ourselves away, to let nature run rabid.

The river,
the goose,
the forest
know more than we how to let go,
to linger in the magical

transience without firming grips on the
control panel that is
not at their discretion
to manipulate.

Perhaps we only learn how to let go
as I did through brute force—
by movement eclipsed that robbed me of knowledge
I misunderstood for the
skeleton of the universe,
by being immobilized in the cast of grief,
by the immense weight of loss.

A refugee,
I was suddenly evicted out of my own body,
my own life—
an unfortunate paradigm of parallax—
a nomad wandering the desolate alleys of
naked fear at being
alone in my unhappening.

The bravery to witness
to parallel worlds,
to curl your toes over the precipice of everything
you ever thought,
including all past, present and future
species of selfhood,
with the unfaltering knowing that you
will have to give it all away.

The feat and crumble of being completely human with
   yourself.

Letting yourself alone, even on the bleeding
edge of your own disappearance.

Becoming a panopticon,
an all-seeing portal of humanity and humility,
prepared to hold on,
ready to let it all go.

A telescope for hope

Hope is a reincarnated entity,
a cat with nine lives,
a routine recurrent signpost
on the highway, an esoteric Schrödinger's cat
that dies, or perhaps does not die,
a wad of gum that you chew and store in your cheek,
forget about, chew over.

It is sometimes present, sometimes absent.

Oh, the intimate beauty of my
screeching
asymmetry.

We are tree stumps subsisting on sustenance
from neighbors underfoot who lock
fingers with us in
congenial connectivity.

We are incarnate, cut down,
unaccustomed,
adapting infants once more
and ever so ancient,
decrepit,

but here.

Oh, we are so very here—
so excruciatingly aware,
diminished but
incandescent.

The overflowing waste bin of self-erasure and overwhelm.

The melee of our kinked and crumpled being.

I fail to brush off
belief in the impossibility
of recovery back onto my feet.

The primacy of love in this ruined world.

I am the hot coals of trauma,
the veering tubes
of oxygen feeding my flabbergasted brainstem.

Maybe, one day, hope might
return or might not return, and in that might—
those incalculable statistics,
that perhaps probability—
is adequate sufficiency
in the darkest of days,
during the cruelest hours,
during the most brutal circumstance
that no one can relate to,
that you as a writer
flail to pen into words,
syllables,
cesurae,
song.

We digress from our lives.

I am learning to
admire my own adaptation,
how my mother's charge matches my own,
seeding an invisible wire between us,
underground knowledge cuts in
close to divinity, a hall of mirrors.
We are each other's shadows,
as organic as mist on sea.

I weary, wobbly,
wordless, in these unwalkable
muddy walkways of disability.

I am bound together by what ifs too impossibly
sharp for language, incompressible feeling
so oversized that any attempt to shove it
into cumbersome black and white letters exhausts.

I am an artifact of encroachment,
busy with the overwintering
occupation of survival.

I am a litany of glitches.

My seeing has been
drastically, abrasively, altered,
clipped.

I can no longer create my own conditions.

Can you?

My brain throbs, lurches to disengage
from this revised scale of life—

when the residual details
become mountains too
splendid,
punctuated,
permeated,
with purpose.

This is how I account for myself—
my crash out of my normal,
my tenacity to mount compassion for this form.

I stutter over
this vigilant
unease.

My tragedy hit the dower wrong note in my
nervous system,
throwing me outside of hope's reach.

It is tricky to find hope
in hopelessness,
in bottomlessness,
in a room that is pitch, slanted black
painted over and again in black—-
without lamp light, without windows,
without anything to radiate the world, to set some object
  ablaze.

Let me know if you
find hope and have some to spare.

Sometimes, there is a respite or interlude of silence,
a grace period,
as though you were waiting

in a doctor's office far too long, your scheduled time offset
by the arrival of another patient.

Can you feel the bleeding texture of my world?

The once microscopic aspects of reality have
mushroomed into full bloom under my radar—
small bites of food that I
can taste on the left side of my tongue
grow decadent,
succulent,
a shoulder dislocation from
my threadbare connective tissue
more devastating,
more gruesome,
more complicated,
due to my utter lack of self-knowledge of this body absent
of sensation on the denigrated right.

I am losing every day.

I am losing the day,
and the day is losing me.

The loss that weighs down most upon my spirit
is that of self-awareness—
my former outrageous repository
gone.

I could once foretell as limbs emerged from sockets,
put the pieces of my body back together.
I could tidy up my mess of self before it spilled out of hand.

I am at an impasse with my right side,
fighting hard each day for basal function.

I am homesick for myself.

Are you?

I miss my hope in myself.

I do not need
quantum physics, genetics, linear algebra or
any of the studies I once
thought paramount to my
excelling in the world,
but I do need to know myself.

I do need to know my body.

I do need to know
where the right side of me is,
where the right side of the
world starts and I end.

I am looking to find my way through this
fractured night to some light,
however dim,
to some hope,
however faint,
to some inner knowing,
however incomplete,
that might still be
mine or might not be
if something,
anything,
changes.

Come alive with me

This world has always been a mind away, the funnel of focus extracting receptive pleasure, the sunlight from awareness. It is only since my body has been mangled and crippled that I have come to acknowledge its unparalleled wisdom and indomitable beauty. The fleeting nature of being can be drawn closely only when our lives slam against a hard and unforgiving corner— when our breath is almost leached out of us. Mine almost faced a final period. Now, I will never again surrender to ignorance of the body's majestic and cryptic intelligence.

But what about water? Does it too expire? Perhaps there is some-thing vibrating with life on this Earth that never dies. Perhaps that is the ultimate resting place for the soul. I long to blunt the spears of my mind clawing their way towards a desire for death over this liminality—this disabled body unsuited for this world.

What if I permit my body to speak to me in its own poetic rapture of doing and then go on a word search inside my mind, to let the silent elegance of my faulty yet enduring form lead me from the night well into the sunlight, to forgo causal relationships we label explanations and simply open like the petals of a flower into being? The superpower of my disability is that I can now feel time. I can now hear through my skin. I can now hear the soft sonata of breath, the sea of my being that catches me over and again. I can now feel emptiness as a presence, a webbing to everything. I just have to exhale and extend my spine upward to touch that distant pine, to be one with stars. I am learning how to occupy space again, how to flex my relationship with gravity through micro-movements of my torso, noticing that my physical collapse is not a fait accompli, that I am still capable of expansion, of inflating skyward.

Do you believe that there is something alive in the quiet emptiness of your body? My body, even the half of it I misremember, whispers its narrative to me in its own adolescent vernacular. I must learn to listen, to become attune to a foreign frequency. I must lend my ears more patience.

What is the story in your body? You must find it, not with your eyes pointed outward, but with your gaze angled inward—your external eyes bounded into blindness, or into a different type of internal sight—into the pillar of your being.

How else can you arrive at your midline?

There is remarkable complexity in this simple task. In this space of internal vision, I discover the skin on my fingertips, how to feel it course through my whole body, how to let the light in, how to assert myself out of the stagnant echo in my mind—the reverberating plea to yield to my will's desire to exit this life, this malicious malignancy of being marginalized in a body no longer fated to walk, to independence.

My body is infinitely more certain than my mind in its contention to live. My body is infinitely wiser than my will in its aptitude to heal, to bring me back to center over and again, even though my midline, my spinal cord, is now where my right side ends inside my mind. My mind does not know everything. My body knows better, better than anything in this world. I beseech my body to help me find my riverbanks again—to help me locate the boundaries between me and the right side of the world.

We often fail to recognize the simplicity harvested within the matrix of the world—how, for instance, the ratio of large to small trees in a forest is rooted in a fractal, how an arboreal communion is based in nature's mellifluous mathematics, not in our own. Why does the mind strive over and again to overshadow and to smother the silent brilliance of the body?

Perhaps, I can be in the happening instead of dwelling in the interior of my mind, narrowing the distance between me and the world, even when the physical world and my physical body in this shadowland feel irreconcilably out of phase.

Perhaps I can believe in the subtle swaying of my trunk
    and feel
the inklings of a smile creep along my mouth,
so life eventually presses down on me a bit more gently, so
    that I can grow
out of the straitjacket of my mind
that clings to the wound,
to this seismic sense of an
ending at what should have been
the beginning of my life.

A Denison of Saturn

I wait for the words to dribble,
gentle awakening rainwater,
to tie themselves about my tongue past parted lips.

Oh, these beauteous but thoroughly inadequate
leaky blankets of lines and contours,
blunt spears of noise intervening silence roped together
    into what we deem coherency.

We, mortal and breaking beings, fashioned this alphabet.

If only nature, that flawless generator,
constructed this construct,
then perhaps the lived experience of disability
could be enfranchised, embodied, erupt into full-throttled
   being inside this
black and white refuge, this now verbal cage.

For no matter how prolonged the necklace of words,
the incalculable depths of my disability—
the how and why I choose my body over no longer
   being—
can never be stenciled on the notecard of language.

And yet, I await the words and beam
at their advent,
as though I were a plant awaiting sunrise, its delivery of
   nutrients.

For they remain my singular currency to counter trauma's
   encroachment,
its fastidious foreclosure on my neatly packaged three
   decades.

I am unscrewed from the machine of my life,
living beneath the agonizing specter of was.

The script of this present existence—
who authored it?

Who edited it and unleashed it for publication?
For even dreams have been snagged, a rug tearing at its
   fringes,

disfigured, adopted the dystopian outlines.

Perhaps this is radical acceptance.

Perhaps this is a surrender of my armor, submission to the
    turbulence of mortality.

Perhaps this is dysphoria of the soul as it falls.

The content and demographic of my dreams remains
    unaltered, unadapted to my after,
but I have been gruesomely tailored—
my physical body pared back to match my current form
    welded to formlessness.

And the fear would perhaps slenderize if I were no longer
gallivanting through Harvard Yard,
serving a tennis ball to my father,
swerving beneath a mighty tide,
sauntering across New York pavements as I mentally
solved linear algebra problems
into now revolting resolution.

Because I am
stripped of two vital quadrants
that once made me whole.

15 months into the gaping void of my trauma,
my dreamscape depicts my body shorn of my entire right
    side.
I am but half of me,
as I am in the devastation,
the Great Depression,
of my reality that empties the pockets
of my soul,

that still feels unreal,
that may always feel surreal,
that may always render me a denizen of Saturn.

What about Earth?

What about my place on Earth?

But I am still waiting for the words, because despite their
    fledgling inadequacy,
they are my only mode of transportation beyond,
or maybe through, the locked gates of despair and
    incredulity
into a place resembling peace,
a contained variety of quiet,
a control mechanism on the wheels
tensioning me hastily into somber disrepair,
however faulty and porous a means of holding
this broken tabernacle in their palms.

I will let them be the tether on which I will tug and tug
    until I reach shore—
lifelines I dictate in lines, shadows of frostbitten flickers.

Because yes,
there is immense pain,
irretrievable should-have-beens.

But what else is there?

There is a remapping of my mind as it learns to dance
    again with my now
irreconcilable spinal cord.

There is a letting go of anger towards this body that tastes
  like betrayal.

But that is the voice inside my head.

My body aches to be here.

There is an unlearning of the classroom
knowledge I presumed my license for existence.

There is learning how to harness
the reserve of energy I never lost
and never before found that I leverage
to land in symmetry,
even when my physicality lives off-balance,
to locate the warm soft light within that no
trauma can switch off,
that only I can dial into when I become conscious of
my breath breathing me
into becoming.

There is the remarkable fertility of suffering
from which I will sprout
into someone I know not yet,
aside from the bare fact
that she remains grateful
for what still remains.

Conclusion

The poems in this section transcribed the constant pain and
confusion caused by the speaker's stroke, which reflected,
through shifting narrative and time jumps, the way that trauma
pulls sufferers back and forth in temporal space. Writing pieces

of her story keeps the speaker alive. Analyzing and deepening her understanding of her new reality becomes the only way to keep going.

Movement II
Stasis

Introduction

In this section, the speaker is conflicted between a yearning to resuscitate her early years in Memphis, Tennessee, and to forget the memories that haunt her. The speaker's loss of feeling and awareness of the right side of her body motivate her to open lines of discourse with this half of herself and the complications of her genetic connective tissue disorder. She grapples for a semblance of equilibrium between what was and what is, between what she senses and no longer senses, between the margins' liberation and restriction.

Penumbra

I host a vigil for this borrowed life,
sifting through the grime of what is still preserved in the
    prism of memory.

My shadow blinks into near darkness.
Come find me.

My past is a stowaway in the bowels of my mind, a
    penumbra—
a partial eclipse, a but semi-shadow blurring at the corners
    as time overtakes me,

tramples me out of my former life.

Let me recall what was.

Do not let it all bleed out.

My stroke took enough, right?
But is enough ever enough?

I have vacated myself, lights diminishing on my body's
    vigor.

I grow archaic and arcane as dread kneads into a knot in
    my trachea,
occluding my already impeded oxygen—
once only a beatific element on the periodic table,
now a vital constituent my body struggles to strain out of
    air—
the insufferable reminder ringing, a persistent bell, that I
    am the evidence,
the excavated ruins, the lead in my own tragedy, in the
    stronghold of strife.

I forfeit this but piecemeal shadow of being.

Set me free, world.

If only this stroke
would unfold into a chess board I could overcome with
    strategic logic,
with a calculating mathematical mind once a key to every
    door—
my passport to excel, to outsmart existence.

But the world is no such patina—there is no opening
    gambit to play,

no reasonable game boxed with intact pieces that yield to
    deduction.

Instead, life cracks open,
and I fell into its barbed crevice.

Light flickers into darkness, into night.

A savage misstep-
this bewailing brainstem, this receding flash of reality.

I need this penumbra of being to crackle into light,
into blinding exposure, to acquire the sublime equilibrium
    of water rising and falling its way home.

What is home?
Remind me as I forget.
Do not force me to forfeit my shadow altogether.
Do not rend me into more fragments that crumble,
    granules in my fist.

Let me leave some footprints behind, not just a penumbra,
so that you will one day find me, so that you are not left
    alone.

Permit me to watch the world go as white as a blank page
    with snow,
and let me leave my footfalls behind, even if I cannot feel
    the sole of my right foot.

I do not fear my fragmented shadow—
the right side of my body I don't perceive.

This unshakable cotton silence of solitude,
these feeble weapons of words bandaged in the gauze of
    painful yearning.

Penumbra—
let me flee my penumbra in this after.

Let me be that orb of light unextinguished.
Let me be that tangle of limbs again,
that innocent ear enlivened by melodies with volume that
    hurts.

Let that be the only flavor of pain pervading my being.

Let me kiss the ground in sheer relief at being human-
a dancing creature dripping with luminous energy,
a body radiating love that is only acquainted with
    penumbra in abstraction,
not as an embodied essence seeping through the surface
    of my skin.

Do not let me drift off.

Not yet, world.

Not yet.

Let me hold time at bay, so I can start to catch up with
    myself.

Add one more day, one more minute,
one more second, to my before.

I keep fighting for the impossible.

What does it feel like to lose a soul?

Have I felt that already?

But we are all forever unready to look across the street
    from our own ending.

Who wants to trail off?

But, here, in this after, I am starting to learn that I can
locate my own inner light source, so I can begin to paint
    the missing outline
of my form- the lost part of my penumbra—
making something excruciatingly fragile but wonderful,
    nonetheless,
in this ending, this disjuncture, this almost start.

Here I go, remembering who I was, looking out towards
    who I can become,
threading fingers through pinkies of time until past and
    future spill into each other,
a watercolor blooming with eternal vitality.

Phantom limb

The phantom limb of this loss and pain are unlike imaginary friends who once swelled my consciousness with unassailable smiles and innocent secrets, refusing to exit my psyche at the dinner table or on the swing set, leaving me perfectly at ease in my own uneasy solitude. My spinal cord and brain injury are more like meteors hammering permanent indentations on my raw body and inside my mind, cracking me, paring me back to the basics, and lurching me backward—a blitzing time travel out of maturation.

The grief is elusively translucent, uncatchable by any effort to pin it down hard and fast, to look at it with eyebrows raised and request its departure date. Your prayers, however well-intentioned and impassioned, will not mend my stroke. Trust me, words do not harbor that incantatory lure we compel them to. We are human prey. Too often, we forget we are animals—not altogether divergent from that robin or wren.

This phantom limb pain does not come with the expiration date of imaginary friends, nor with an outgrowing. But it does not occlude a growing outward, an arabesque of mind. For, I have learned that this emptiness in my soul, this void in my disabled body, is not only empty but is also full. Full of what, I have yet to discover, or, perhaps, to invent, to trip my way back into child-hood reveries. I may always live with this phantom limb—this exaggerated, exasperating urgency to become the girl pre-served in my before, the girl who strikes me as incredulous, as a phantasm.

But I will fill myself up again. But I will settle into the empty spaces within, with the phantom limb of loss and suffering inking scars on my spirit that gush and ooze with a crimson beyond the visi-ble spectrum. I will look upon them as touchstones to be grateful for every blessing of still being someone whose trauma could have been her last breath.

Reader, squeeze my hand a bit harder into yours.
I am not that delicate.
I can take it.
I need it.
Let me feel you remembering me,
remembering you.

Tending to my living death

Why must we wait for our pulses retire to eulogize our
  lives,
to knit syllables to empty space into the book report of
  self,
if to live entails coping with a small portion dying
along the way?

I have become food-splotched and threadbare
dolls from my childhood, literally coming unglued, my
  parts an orchestra
with an absent-minded conductor.

My right shoulder contorts to its
own staccato out of joint.

My right hip dislocates
to a discordant falsetto.

My right ribs—
the fingers of my nervous system—
are limber piano keys
falling into disrepair in the delicious slumber of night
crackling with shuddering bursts of excruciating
  unanchoring.

My mother cradles my right arm into socket with what
  feels
like duct tape in preparation for shipment to a foreign
  country.

My body—
this entity so robustly unaccustomed to me—

packaged in a wheelchair
in the rear of a car
is more like human cargo
than a human being,
an outmoded model of our species
ready for exchange, ready for novelty, ready to become the
    next generation of self.

I do not expect myself to ever fully absorb
the shock of my loss—
my zest for biology, for thrusting my hand into the air
to answer academic questions neatly paved with solutions,
for propelling myself through math problems and novels,
for gliding through glistening grass as I observed nature
    uncork itself.

This girl embarking on her PhD in genetics
is buried beneath the soil in my soul,
and I visit her internally when the blade of grief stabs me.

Yet my heart still beats.

Yet the grass still grows.

Yet the world still happens
with me, without me.

And I wonder
how this happening
is still happening.

I intuit that to live in this world means holding hands with
    death.

So the question spirals,

a broken record inside my mind,
as to why we only commemorate
the dead when the living are dying too-
when we carry several lives past within us
we often fail to recognize,
let alone to memorialize.

I wish I could whisper the Judaic Kaddish
for that previous version of myself—
for that girl unmade
by my spinal cord stroke.

The tears for her are a river.

I hold her—
a dead baby kangaroo
in the pouch of my right side
I can neither feel nor control.

Maybe she lingers in this empty space.

Maybe she fills it.

Who is to say what happens when this undefinable thing
   we call I dies
yet our bodies continue to persist?

So I will bring her roses.

So I will tend to her gravesite.

So I will live as she dies.

I will endeavor to remember her smiling gaze,
her love affair with existence,
her unquenchable thirst for knowledge.

I will become
a citadel,
a shrine,
a coffin
for this person I treasured being.

But I will simultaneously become someone as I adapt and
    survive,
despite the crushing cataclysm of being-
the onslaught of pain and grief-
because here I am—
whistling in the dark,
palpating the world with my right hand
that no longer perceives sensory input,
courageously confronting today in these words,
in this thicket of silence,
emerging out of weeping soil,
a tree uprooted that still,
in defiance of logic,
branches skyward,
however gradually,
however broken and incomplete.

About-Face

Squint with razor-sharp force until it hurts, and it could be me.
I could be you. Neglect all of the negligible heritable assets of
hue and contour. Forget everything except for the naked bones
that delineate a life. See that woman right there pushing a
stroller. See that infant holding her mother's palm. See that girl
with a tawny bun texting while consuming a morning muffin on
her commute to an office. See that student in a lab coat zooming

down Lexington Avenue with a microscope in hand. See that haggard woman, her eyes coated with a sleepless glaze, six or nine months pregnant, a tense band of skin exposed between her top and pants. See that cohort of 20-somethings participating at ear-smothering decibel levels in that highly underrated, sacred juggling act of walking and talking. I want to scream. I desperately need to throw something somewhere, anything anywhere. All of the potential that was once my molecular composition, my capstone, my inner resources, has crashed out, spilled over the brim into a pandemonium of seeping frantic kinetic energy. But, to everyone beyond the threshold of my skin, nothing at all, whatsoever, has transpired. Everything marshals forward, arrows pointing in progress' direction. I am decaying as I live, yet the world fails to take notice—as though I was never in its warm generous and generative center to begin with, as though I had no balustrade from which to fall. I am locked inside of a nervous system shocked by my ongoing phantasm in this afterword. I am zapped, accosted by too much scrutiny, too much watching other lives unfold while mine is caught in the lattice of still motion, ember in the in-between. My coming out into the world slipped, backflipped into a coming in—into what I am not yet sure. There are so many questions that slosh around my brain that I am too terrified to put words to, to hear the English translation of that which I am not yet primed to touch, to feel simmer in syllabic arcs. I have been discharged of the duty of being Elly, in enforced transit from a defined active participant to an amorphous anthropologist, observing the world from a far-away anonymous place from which there is no exit. Squint with immense intent, and it could, I could, be anyone. We could be occupying opposing roles on the stage set that is the world and that the world sets. You think you can be anything. You yearn to trudge up a workaround for my scenario. Unfortunately, this is implausible, out of bounds of being human. You think you have all the time in the world. But, my dearest reader, we all run dry, and we are swiped blank. I was you. We soar, but how briskly and suddenly we drop. We can be at both poles, holding up the bandwidth of the tent of our species so that we are all seen for everything we are, everything we can no longer become.

Apocalypse

A catastrophe of biblical proportions, an implosion of self.
I am lost in translation with myself, caught in the labyrinth
    of pain, of time losing its momentum and slipping, as
        though the clock took off its shoes and risked its way on
        socks across newly varnished wood.
Thoughts of genetics and mathematical proofs—
once my fertile soil and my firmament—
no longer steady me as the floor buckles under a right foot
    I no longer sense.
Tell me, amnesia of my soul quickening, what hope and
    freedom feel like in disability.
Tell me over and again, until the drum beat of your words
    percusses against my chest.
I need your language to catch me as I fall.
Events slide out of order, growing fuzzy and hazy at their
    periphery,
stacks of clothing unfolding themselves.

Logic no longer adheres in this hell.

I am someplace beyond the boundaries of my expertise-
metamorphosing from scientist to specimen-
in desperate need of a permission slip to belong
  somewhere, anywhere, as my reference, my compass,
  demagnetizes, malfunctions, misdirects.

I am a satellite, a UFO, a misfire of your consciousness—
a stroke shedding me of myself,
ripping away the settings of underdeveloped adulthood
  from my becoming.

The vernacular of my body—
a seen language, a ledger, an audit, an entire bookcase of
  plots
I yearn to worm my way out of but have no other skin to
  inhabit.

The right half of me redacted of awareness is a map of
  bruises
punctuated by lacerations as ribs, a hip, an elbow nudges
  their way out of joint,
my connective tissue disease unveiled in all of its entoptic
  gory by this apocalypse.

I wear fear in tight latitudes across my forehead.

My gaze glazes over.
I withdraw ever further into myself.

I am a tree uprooted.
All that remains are sharp branches.

I limp against my innate nature,
stung by the needle of trauma, as I try to locate a web of
  being,

shorn of the ligaments and tendons that once forged me
   into function and structure.

I yearn for my own diseased connective tissue to glue me
   back into the socket of self,
to resuscitate me out of this apparition of a life, this
   dislocation of being, this falsified smile that but emerges
   at the absurdity of my rupture-
a body at the mercy of a right side that no longer synapses
   me into a beautiful creature besotted by embedding
   itself in rainstorms, in fields of wild grasses
I could once tread upon and sense with ease, a physical
   form that was once so right it
felt translucent, so light and luminous, so tender and
   devoted to intellect—
to fathoming the world through rigid rubrics of science, to
   analyzing my
way through Tolstoy or Bach concertos.

Where did all of those reasonable rudiments go?

I do not care if I misapprehended the world for a causal
   microcosm—
I will take my former delusion over this brutal, biting truth.

I live within nuanced expressions, trapped in ember by this
   tragedy too outsized for
mundane words that crop it into something too curt for its
   endless depths.

I yearn to depart from these ghosts I carry, children I will
   never carry, this restrained,
silenced apocalyptic existence howling, a wild beast
   ensnared.

I cry alone and in chorus with all other soft mortally broken
    and breakable organisms sobbing in this very instant.

In each moment, we are mourning and enduring—
feeling blessedness for what lingers and flinging our
    disabled bodies to our knees,
begging the cosmos for all we can no longer long for.

If only memory were more like an archive, time-lapse
    video footage I could continually revisit without its
    details fraying, smudging into oblivion.

Do you know that you are right here, a respiring fleeting
    composite of frail skin and bone?

Caught in the crossfire of my reeling body, my brain
    starves for a taste of control,
however illusory, now only realizable in these small Latin
    rooms,
stanzas, as I find new rhetoric, rhythm and meter.

I let go of tense sadness that pulls me under my own feet
    in
these stanzas, and transform into an interior decorator-
I furnish and carpet these rooms with emotions chanting
    in my soul,
string mirrors along walls so I begin to become acquainted
    with myself,
tread delicately on threadbare rugs and creaking
    floorboards paneled
with wood that splinters at intervals,
shocking the sole of my left foot leftover,
string curtains that refuse to entice sunlight, as I loop to
    nowhere

along their perimeter, my breath falling rough and jagged
as tears slam into these stanzas,
onto the white of this page.

I could protest against this version of my life through
   hours,
but I opt to chisel these stanzas,
to stencil the shape of a soul I seek to birth,
because this apocalypse could have been my death,
and in too many ways, it jettisoned my matrix of self and
   time,
but it did not end me.

So I will be the interior designer
of these stanzas of soul and procreate myself into
someone who can neither unlearn nor unhear
all of the thrashing loss but who can still
become infatuated with being here-
someone mortal and shuddering who can hear
the birdsong overhead, crane her neck heavenward,
and be enraptured with the nature that permeates each
   moment.

For even when we feel irreparably alone,
unsalvageable vagabonds in navy night of life,
we never truly are.

Dandelions on tombstone

She broaches the tombstone, tremulous yet cherubic,
a blonde veil of ringlets
simmering in October breeze.

Her red glistening Mary Janes scatter majestic ruby dust
amidst the ashes and gravel
crunching underfoot—
melting memory, desire, the death of innocence.

Her blue jumper and fistful of dandelions define her,
coalesce her into a profound pantheist.

She is a Russian doll incarnate,
a thrumming heart replete with unchecked euphoria,
desolate of all the pain
reality will brand upon her soul.

Time collapses in upon itself,
a 1950s fan women held.

Nothing is past.

Nothing is yet to come.

Everything is right now,
in the open palm of this moment.

She is at once an infant crashing into the world,
and a 28-year-old whose life took a turn
for the worse,
a stroke deserting her in the desert of lost creatures,
left her wondering what was left other
than her left side.

She sees time as a strange loop,
swirling in upon itself, the convolution of all that
has happened, will happen
or unhappen.

She realizes that nothing ever dies,
that she is mourning for someone both
gone and here, perhaps permeating
the very molecules of air entering her nostrils.

And yet, she is still visiting herself-
her shadow, her subterranean ghost
buried in a lab coat and clutching a pipette, readying
   herself
postmortem to inoculate a vial of cells.

I yearn to give my five-year-old self a hug,
to tell her to grab hold tightly to her once seemingly
infinite wad of innocence, to tell her that she will be
alright at not being
all right.

I yearn to whisper into her ear that she must keep going,
no matter what the world does
to jostle her upside down, to capsize her everything.

She places dandelions on her future tombstone, as though
   she were
donating some of her innocence in advance of her
   avalanche,
some of her golden beatitude for the world to the light
   that
has been depleted,
that will be eclipsed,
from her much older
and far too wise self to be.

She thinks the dandelions are a panacea.

Let's let her think that.

She thinks she can immunize her all too soon
debilitated self that all she must do is cling to nature
and the rest of reality will just right itself like an upset
  stomach.

But she will not have a broken leg.

She will not even have cancer.

She will have an entire life, an entire future,
ripped so hastily, and without warning, from her.

She will have everything that matters to her abstracted
  away,
as though her entire life were drawn with a crayon
on gravel that has been effaced by time and scrubbing.

Even this four-year-old girl mourns herself, and what she
  does not know is coming.

She wants to scream at the universe for capturing her
  innocence
as she once captured caterpillars and lightning bugs.

But even this four-year-old girl knows how to grieve.

She will learn that for her grieving and living must go
  hand-in-hand.

She will learn the game of hide and seek she once
adored she will soon despise
as she will have to play with herself without end,
as she will be on a ruthless and exasperating search for the
  right side of her body

and will never find its hiding place.

But, for now, a year has passed since she was struck in her
    brainstem and spinal cord
and all the four-year-old girl can do is deliver dandelions.

Sometimes there are no words.

Sometimes there is not even a tombstone.

Sometimes there are only memories that touch each other
    through the bandwidth
of time to let you know that you will be,
that you might be,
enough.

Somatic intelligence

The voice of suffering is declarative thunder.

I am trying to teach myself out of the morass of trauma
    that
overwrites and undoes me over and again through replay
    of memories,
acquiring dimensionality and scale that shrink me into a
    microcosm of self.

My right side speaks to me in muted whispers,
in hushed vapors of wordlessness—
a song of scarred silence,
a presence of absence, gravitational burdens experienced
as leaden weight mounted to my torso.

I have transgressed the human form, evolved or devolved
    into a species unmade for this planet,

but unwilling to shirk the enduring gentle courage to
    endure.

My right side hums a foreign melody,
a somatic intelligence.

It does not require syllables strung together into
    something resembling sensibility.

Do we ever truly make sense?

Do words ever weave us into the textured tapestry of
    humanity?

Perhaps we are more understood in vast pauses, in the
    preverbal softness of trees.

My right side carries its own tune, especially as night darts
    blackness through sky.

This is when my right half bellows its sonorous and
    resounding symphony of neurons firing,
embodied invisible blasts of fireworks showering my
    confounded brain,
which refuses to communicate with this forsaken,
yet still vital, segment of me.

I have been interrupted from myself.

But my right-side dances to its own unheard music,
    trembling ataxia through the world,
notifying me of its existence in its cottony quiet,
its capacity to rejoice through the rainfall
of my shuddering tears.

My right side is teaching me how to let go—

how to find meaning in intractable stasis,
how to find abundance in scarcity,
how to hum without speech,
how to legitimize myself in this state of precarity,
how to delicately belong inside the
affliction of the unexplained,
how to live within this detour that has
grown into my default,
how to feel without sensation.

I am learning how to converse with
these two quadrants of my body I presumed were forever
    lost to me
by a stroke I initially thought my dead stop that
turned out to be a hasty pivot point-
a stupefying moment of inflection inoculating me with
a hefty dose of sorrow,
but also with superhuman audacity
to become my own shifting paradigm,
to wake to the small fledgling voice in the abyss,
the refuge in the world's recantation of its apparent
    promises.
I am recovering a different species of Eden.
There was once a ravenous need to fill any void with a rush
    of words,
sound I could hear, which I assumed to be the sole flavor
    of noise in this world.

I am learning from my right side that silence is oftentimes
    the opposite of emptiness,
that an absence can be so full of everything we never
    thought possible

because we never had to contemplate
the inextinguishable and inexpressible language of our
  bodies,
their lexicon emergent from apocalypse.

I train my deaf ear to listen close in to the
harpsichord harmonizing in my right interior,
to the mesmerizing melody wired into
the nervous system of every
being that was,
is and will be.

Connective tissue

Connective tissue—
bookbinding of humanity, foundational and fundamental
  glue comprising fragile
lattices of cells stitched to proteins that buckle us into
  becoming, basement membranes upon which layers
  array, gardening us into verdant communion.

Connective tissue—
I am out of joint with my world, with myself, my
  connective tissue enfeebled by disease now a threshold
  transgressed by a stroke of medical malpractice,
a subluxation of self.

Someone staring back in mirrors wears my skin,
the exotic cloaked in native.

Who are you?

Give me back that costume of self, that necessary rubber
  band connecting me to you.

Connective tissue—
I am disconnected from everything that once gathered
    me into being,
atrophying by the day, my vital sheath severed, its
    perimeter serrated as I fall out of myself, out of order, into
    solitary confinement in darkness alongside my disabled
    body—
waiting, moaning, panting—
the too patient patient, for a gush of morning light to
    segregate dawn.

Connective tissue—
I tension at recollections of your invisible embrace, your
    delicate, precious wrapping, desperate to live in the
    connective tissue of these sacrosanct days,
to steady myself once more in the socket of the familiar-
brace myself through brutal winters,
fan my hand through invincible summer suns,
cry bucketfuls of tears with the sky wailing rain,
fold myself like corners of novel pages dogeared to mark
    their poignancy
into this existential pulse, linking my own faulty connective
    tissue to mankind's.

But the inevitable undergrowth of entropy cradling
    through everything
throbbing with life gruesomely altered underfoot,
the external world blitzing out of alignment.

Connective tissue—
I surrender to my departure, to the unfathomable breach
    in my own connective tissue

as limbs and ribs cross Rubicons of sockets on the right
    half of being numb and unaccustomed to my brain
    jolted by this stroke.

I am a first-generation car,
a BlackBerry,
a 1998 computer—
something unbelievably and irrefutably obsolete.

But I am but 28, I want to scream into the void in my heart.

I corral myself into tranquility, a baby kangaroo nuzzling
    into an interior pouch.

Connective tissue—
I thirst for this dislocation out the choreography of my past
to be more like water- a substance that elegantly and
    mellifluously descends while retaining structure.
How does water maintain its beautiful bondage as it falls
    between oxygen and hydrogen atoms without tearing
    wide-open like us?

The mind can only aspire to understand water's duality-
its simultaneous aliveness and immorality, a marvelous
    miracle of Earth's tears,
its never-ending homeostatic dynamic between life and
    death.

Connective tissue—
my physical layout is tarnished,
disjointed from the future once as real as my racing heart-
the almost geneticist cultivating romantic relationships,
almost entwining herself in a love affair with the external
    world,

almost unlocking the gates inside her being so she could
    meld her
own connective tissue with that of the cosmos,
become a spangled being in dialogue with moonlight.

But the blessed reality of all of that is now overwritten
    by the bold typeface of trauma- not even a palimpsest
    leaving a residue-
the connective tissue between me and the world beyond
    my boundaries unspooling, acquiescing to my genetic
    connective tissue disease as though it were a contagion,
    a virus swimming broad strokes through the world,
disenfranchising me of everything I once knew, I once
    thought could be known.

But this world is not a legible read.

Connective tissue—
my right side is no longer right-
no longer laces me together into the seamless map of the
    known,
but it is not wrong either.

It is still here—
however uprooted from my brain, from caressing hands.

Oh, what a painful jog of memory—
that once blessed tactile life curdling to the surface with
    almost painful effervescence.

Connective tissue—
this universe does not yield to human imperatives,
does not grow us connective webs into life anew.

But these words lapping at your ears are growing molars,

forging skin and limbs that walk me beyond the periphery
   of self onto something verging on solid ground.

So, I will let myself land here—
on this white page—
my newfound connective tissue
synapsing me into a new beginning, into dynamic with
   you, as I learn to weave these scorched, jagged pieces of
   my soul into artistic expression.

Threshold

If words are the only vehicle to transgress the threshold of
   skin,
to impart the contents of our essences,
these black cryptic contours do not quench the
urgency to transmit sensory experience,
particularly when circumstances are
paranormal and out-of-step with the drumbeat of
   humanity,
when the torrential downpour of disability
strikes you so particularly that you are the first
to survive the landslide of a medullary
stroke and cervical cord injury mapped onto your
chronic connective tissue disease.

There is a bellowing subliminal undertone buried beneath
   the words,
or between the words that cannot be uttered,
can only be voiced in the silo of self,
a reverberating echo-chamber of desolate aloneness.

But, if these black letters are our only route out of the self, there is a distinction that time and grief elucidate.

There is a critical difference between illness and disability-
between the beauty of the seesaw-like dance between
    the kingdom of the ill
and relative wellness and the lockdown within the
    dystopia of your own skeleton,
those gates into relative health, independence and
    function slammed shut,
impenetrable.

I yearn for the days when words were a melody,
tunes readily picked up by other souls,
when my anomalous reality peppered with routine
    shoulder dislocations
and setbacks but landed me a few steps behind myself,
armed me with the capacity to catch up to myself, to get
    caught up in my world,
to generate a web of a life interrupted by an illness
that did not accost my body like this trauma,
this uprooting of all of my roots so assiduously and
    intricately borne beneath my feet.

I am afraid of hope, more at one with the uncertainty that
    corsets me,
for I am petrified to anticipate the impossible,
to lose more of myself than I already have.

And yet, time elapses, collapsing me into what feels like an
    unexpandable accordion,
bringing about yet another birthday, another year of
    survival depleted of living.

And, for my 29th birthday,

I long to unborn, unfashioned, undone so immaculately
    that I can begin from scratch,
from the kernels of my being,
so that I can dwell within a body that is built for being in
    this world,
for exploring nature, for encountering myself, not just right
    here-
in these dictated words, but in physical form-
in wandering through landscapes, in burying toes I can
    feel in sand,
in being embraced and sensing another's lingering touch
on both sides of my spinal cord,
not just the left side.

I crave to be left alone by feckless, brutal circumstance,
for the stronghold of the shackles on my body to be
    smattered,
for my invisible agony and disrepair to come into full-view
    and then to dissipate altogether.

But I know better than to wish, that doing so only boxes
    me into the victim
status I may deserve but certainly do not desire.

There is nothing triumphant in wedging myself against the
    edge that confines me.

For, if I am to make something of myself beyond simply
    becoming a survivor,
I will not label myself a victim.

Because, despite their inadequacy,

words have a humbling yet penetrating power to tell us
  who we are,
what we are.

I will whisper to myself the story of a heroic girl who found
  solace,
silent suffering, grit and grace in the mire of disability—
a word that may be fastened to her like a belt but that she
  grew into and out from,
becoming something perhaps broken but also capable of
  redemption.

Constellation of scars

There is no wormhole in my mind—
no neural circuitry I can call upon to fire away at the
  wilderness, these sharp hours,
my mushrooming constellation of scars.

My left fingertips masochistically gravitate
towards red tears on my right abdomen,
an almost travel guide for the guideless,
a scattered alphabet of trauma, an insurrection against
  paralysis penetrating my right gut,
against my unmaking in miniature bloody hills that iron
  themselves
into a purpling flatlands of toppling dimensionality,
almost verging into non-existence as they
continue to tell my sweeping saga
of being ripped bit by tiny bit from the landscape of my
  world,
yoking me into a creature branded

with open parentheses,
commas,
blurred 's's and 'o's
swelling with pulse,
tactile truth,
a pointed syncopated synopsis of suffering,
a smattering of lines mapped to nowhere
on my right abdomen.

I am a ship lost at sea,
drifting, shorn of directionality.
Be with me, without a navigator.

These bloody edges
are studded onto the membrane of skin I wear and that
  wears me.

I am a phenix attempting to rise.

My story lives out of focus,
a haze, an entire galaxy swirling with images that spiral out
  of me.

This is how I keep and
save over time—
its wattage,
its current,
its captivity.

I am my own living raw material.

Definitions are losing their value,
slacking into the ill-defined.

What is home?

What is a refuge?

Please let me know if you can carry me to safe ground.

There is nothing left,
save for the words that fester within
I must unfurl to know that I am here,
to know that I have not disintegrated into my stroke,
to know that slivers of my spirit still gravitate towards
    language,
towards a yearning to reverberate in black and white,
towards courage to encounter myself.

I have lost so much that has become indecipherable,
undetectable by verbs and nouns,
by syllables slung together in an effort to make sense of
    nonsense.

Despair overtakes me,
ocean waves at high tide,
my surfboard insufficient to counter
the throttle of water crashing against me,
to counter the fickle nature of good fortune as it gushes
    out of me.

I miss the warm hug of mornings.
I miss the kiss of evening gently dripping across the
    horizon,
that visible, unreachable out yonder.

I wonder how much longer
I can go on this fractured, this scarred.

I am not alone.

Neither are you.

The nested bangles of even the mightiest oak
scarred into the inner sanctum of its trucks, timestamp of
    years,
postage to nowhere,
to everywhere,
a baseboard of notes to self.

At least I have the words to express the malice of the
    world,
the decaying radium of my
should-have-been beginning.

Let us be with each other, with the trees,
tucked between the bedsheets
of white spaces between stanzas.

I have the page and what it can hold,
permitting me to retain a little less grief,
a little less pain,
a little less disquiet.

The page and I share my misfortune.

We are united,
and together we resemble
something testing almost completion.

Negotiating symmetry

If you let me reboot, regenerate, renovate my right side into unity,
into harmony with the rest of me once more, I could be anything.
I could do anything. I would do anything. I would be a garbage

man and carry out your disposal. I might even convert from non-believer to a bonafide disciple of one God or another. You could ask me to do almost anything. You could ask me to change my mind about anything. I would be open to everything, unraveling like pages of an unbound book, because I would have everything I needed and would ever require to dwell on this Earth: two sides of a body interconnected, intertwined, interdigitated. You could ask me to reject all beliefs, to believe in something different, to abnegate all knowledge and possessions, to immigrate to a foreign country, to speak an antiquated tongue, to learn anything, to unlearn everything, to be that woman walking the dogs she does not claim as her own. I could be that adult bagging groceries for which I neither shopped nor desired at the store. I could be that person driving the car to a destination I did not decide upon as a place worth the travel. I would open doors as a doorwoman does for everyone in the world but myself, without asking you for anything, without asking you to say thank you, without even whispering a single word, but a steadying glance, but a soft flash of smile. I would be homeless and find home on street corners, begging no one for money. I would go hungry and cold in winter. I would swelter under the summer suns. I would let leaves fall and gather upon me as summer concludes, seasons churning. I would let the world laugh without asking why, without wondering about anything, without needing anything. I would be a carpenter. I would be a builder. I would be. I would be, if only I could be. I would be fulfilled. I would be loving. I would be worth loving. I am wondering how long it will take me to become whole again, to complete my circuit of selfhood, if completeness is within my realm of expectation in this world, if wholeness is within my reach in this life. If it is not blatantly and brazenly lucid at this point, you should probably quit reading me now or soldier on at your own peril but pause for me to clarify once more. I would be anything. I would just be here in this room in solitude, in breath, in quiet, in morning. I would be at home within myself. I would touch one hand against another and recognize that my right hand was my own, if only my brain could reconfigure its way into this half of me. I would touch one foot against another and notice the contact of skin against skin and own it as something I would never again relinquish. Grant me another chance. Permit me to tether myself into unity; permit me a brief respite of repose, of naked communion with myself, of mildly more obscure humanity, of utter symmetry because right now, in this moment, being half human, being half whole, half here is not enough.

Conclusion

Shedding her fear of revisiting memories of the world before her stroke, the speaker rewinds time to revisit her childhood and explore how to define her survival. While she doesn't come to a particular conclusion, she is able to see the beauty in the past with tenderness and even moments of joy. Writing has become her way of attempting to unify all aspects of herself—past with present, right side with left.

Movement III
Palpitations

Introduction

The speaker comes to a new sense of relationship with her disability. Through her poetry, she interrogates her persistent pain and illness, interrupting her sorrow with satire about her physical predicament. Again, she hungers to piece together the girl she was, but now her language reaches into what is, tying metaphysics and physics into her journey towards acceptance.

Entropy

The tendency of all things to bend in the direction of
    disorder,
a throbbing pulse coincident with the Big Bang 14 billion
    years ago
a nugget of pure energy, nebulous nuclei screaming,
    mayhem muffled beneath the smooth smokescreen of
    constants and integrals, our faltering attempt
to orchestrate chaos into fenced mathematical terms, to
    measure the immeasurable.

A domino somersaulting precipitating its neighbors'
    demise,
a contagion of the soul disseminating into a universal
    pandemic of

pure pandemonium, an image dissolving into the
   unseeable
precisely at the moment of eye contact,
the search for the seamlessness within the infinite sea of
   seams sparking
through the stratosphere, a glass plate striking solid
   ground and shattering without end, the breaking eternal
   without a breaking point to mark its completion.

Entropy—
Earth's expansion engulfs us evermore in this maddening
   tide of all towards disorder.

Entropy—
I am a galaxy a billion light years away from myself.

We are all but oscillating quantum clouds of electrons
   without causality, only probabilistic in our hunger for
   order.

Entropy—
I fell through a pothole in the cosmos, entropy rescinding
   my life, as though I were
but an application.

We hide within bunkers of routine, engage in undying
   liaisons with the illusion of
control as we sort mail, arrange books on shelves,
compose this very stanza, organize rooms and imbue
   structure into our worlds
while cheating on truth rinsing through the cosmos- a
   deafening silence we do
anything to elude, an uncreated, unbound irrationality

too unwieldy for the mind, too unplumbable for the
psyche.

But, unlike the mystified mind, the soul does not
demand solutions, a calculator, an equality nor even an
estimation.

Entropy—
our finite brains fail to compute the infinite, to array this
errant disarray.

But entropy finds us all eventually.

I want to go back to the start, to the quantum Big Bang,
or to graft just part of my before onto this species of
existence.

The soul is sequestered in silence.

It is there waiting for you to find it.

Entropy—
the ungluing of our lives, the hazy softening of edges of
memory at age 28.

In this fire-lit cave of my spirit, I am no longer indigenous
to myself, repopulated in the frail fragrance of trauma, I
decay, a radium of a life-
the once warm embrace of entropy in physics classrooms
infiltrating my core-
my uprooting from laboratory science, physics classes,
dates on calendars and with peers- an entropic hailstorm
that blots me out of myself.

I am sailing away.

Come find me.

Entropy—
If only this stroke were but a bout, a cold, a passing rupture
    of immunity, a fever of sadness soon to break me back
    into the person of my before.

Even my hippocampus, the seat of memory, is not
    inoculated against entropy.

I forget myself.

I drip out of myself more in each moment.

Help me recall who I was, who I was supposed to become.

Entropy—
the dart of time pressing us ever onwards is rooted, posits
    Stephen Hawking,
in the acceleration of entropy, a force he could feel as his
    body unraveled.

Organisms organize, our absurd attempt to counter the
    inevitable
thermodynamic thrust.

We are mortal quixotic miracles of the moment of pattern
    and architecture,
structured of soft flesh and pathways that burgeon and
    dissipate into the atoms in
stars that originated us into ourselves, Darwin's "endless
    forms most beautiful…being, evolved."

Entropy—
perhaps our only purpose in this life is the fruitless
    endeavor to curb entropy, to tighten the lid on a jar that
    will never be sealed.

What about dignity?

I have given in to the cosmic breaking of everything.

Now, in this formless form of life, I let go of the illusion of
   control, the dial that was never intended for fingertips,
   bowing my head in prayer pose to entropy, to the
ruthless dispersal of everything that dilates this moment
   into an unbearably precious sacred stream of seconds.

Do not let them pass by.

I find graceful beauty in unsung melodies splitting silence, in unbreakable corners of words, and in shapes whose contours I am befriending. I am learning that there is elegance in the dependence of disability, that I never was nor am alone because these words, like my ramshackle body at 28, are dependent on the spaces between them, on the emptiness of the white page to nestle against them. As they grow out of the wandering shards of my soul, I am developing with them, cultivating a penchant for entropy—a source of solace that enriches me with the sense of my own ending, cranking wide-open the urgency to commence.

Sonnet minus Iambic Pentameter for my right side

I find myself stewing by the window now, stapled into a fixed posture for hours—head snug between open hands, assuming the hunched contemplation of a mourner. Still, there is no descriptor for me: this almost-dead living entity, this being dangling between two words, neither of which she can negotiate nor absent herself. I sanction myself to tread thoughts of where you, right side, have gone, with the sardonic intent to spin some of this into banter, if only for myself, because without comedy, this tragedy would devour me before breakfast. I posit that you are perhaps on a safari in Africa exploring flora and fauna, cruising through mountain ranges and fields of evergreen, have taken refuge in California or somewhere choked by sunrise. Tell me you find yourself on beaches where my feet can no longer carry me. Tell my imagination to keep darting its indomitable whip around the world, thinking its way into lulling, culling mediations unrealizable. Perhaps you are still here—in this very room affixed to this very body—yet playing the quiet game I once played as a child, refusing to budge. Do you taste the dense fog of silence suffusing everything, taxing each breath? Is that your unaccustomed signature scent—your wordless, dumbfounding presence?

Part of me wonders if part of you mourns for what you and I have lost—the bridge collapsed between us—for the reader who scans these words, this outrageously aggrieved yet romanticized epistle to a cross-section of me at a crossroads with my brain. And if so, I am curious about the texture of your tears. Do they have a color, a pattern, an angle of preferred falling? Do you feel neglected, abstracted, like I do, into the canvas of molecules? You may have severed ties with my consciousness, with the organ of my direct sensory experience—my now impeachable spinal cord—but you, paradoxically, remain fully here in your vacuity, an untamable hunger impossible to shun. In fact, far from being eradicated, you are more intensely felt to me than you ever were when my life was in full bloom. For, to contain you beneath the microscope of my attention—the only scientific apparatus relegated to disabled shores—I concluded I must dilate thresholds of the possible until they have been breached, become more capacious in circumscribing what it means to be a human being. This is to temper, or, rather, to smother, my focus on forward propulsion, on directionality, in pursuit of becoming attune to the surrounding vibrational field. So I spread myself horizontally, a mortal jam, to inscribe you within awareness' arms.

In spite of the waterfall of loss, or, perhaps, because of it, I am my mental stage-setter. The skydiving trip I trust each time I encounter you, my dear right side, once petrified me into the option of abandoning you. But, after the tumultuous wreckage of the past 14 months, I no longer shirk the perplexing feeling of my own collapse when you are right under me, when you were the balustrade holding me erect the whole time. Your former self may have been kidnapped from me, just as my previous manuscript has been abducted, but I will keep seeking your hereness in your negation. I am not on a search for answers. I know what you are thinking—how an unElly of me to no longer throb and pulse to know every intricacy of that biological pathway, that historical detail. But life has been remarkably lite on questions, let alone on answers, in this tense recoil. I am simply a quester of something perhaps tangentially related to hope. Is that the right word? Is there a right word? I do not believe the object of my endeavor is possible or paramount to delineate. The massive value rests in the act of seeking, a task that elevates me above this debris. You see, reader, I regret to inform you that we are all losing our way, losing ourselves along our way. This is life—an unavoidable, but too often underestimated, admixture of vitality and dissolution.

My spinal cord stroke only distilled this truth, an image transitioning from pixilated to incredibly, unbearably, focused that my eyelids snap shut and sigh at regular intervals. I want to learn from you, my darling right side, from your patient grace as you surf—here yet not, alive yet unfelt, functional but dependent on my eyes to locate you. I vow to never stop gesturing to you in our nonverbal code, to never let you go more than you have already gone. If this is not prayer braided into promise, reader, let me know what is and I will edit this text until time runs out.

Interred in now

It is tempting to peer over the wall of this instant, to sneak
  a preview of what lays
in wait in the adjacent room,
a peek into corridors downstream cascading into next
week or even into next year.

There is a plan, we tell ourselves.

I am the master of my own destiny, you like to think.

I coordinate what does or does not occur—how I schedule
  my life,
how I array the layered sediment of years
allotted to me on this planet.

But the room of this instant is often abandoned with hasty
  neglect.

I am contraband, incarcerated within now—
simultaneously captivated, captive, enraptured,
tortured and embraced in

this very moment.

The very next one scares me and the word tomorrow
sliding across my mother's tongue—
lightning scorching my soul.
If only we could project ourselves back onto the walls of
  our befores,
iron the terror running wild in our eyes, injuries raiding our
  spinal cords,
our brains, our territory whited out into a dark thick quiet
  buzzing with everything
now absent.

I am raided of the right half of my body,
the right half of my world—
a partial view,
decimated,
halved.

If you glance in the bullseye of my face,
I will neglect the right half of yours—
left to my imagination,
to my left side,
to my battered brain
to confabulate,
to tabulate into a tableau of your expression.

The yawning space between the girl who left home on
  October 24th
and the girl who returned from the hospital-
immeasurable,
indescribable,
impossible.

I can no longer outline, even in pencil, what may happen
   next.

Can you?

I am strangled within the tense arms of this very breath,
   this very footfall,
this very painful step forward and that insensate one.

I have lost almost everything aside from
what resides within
the four walls of this stanza.

My run-on bucket list once filled with
a PhD, a marriage proposal, children,
traveling the globe, and, above all else,
functional independence.

Against my own will, my list has dissolved,
cruelly tossed aside and cremated.

Nothing remains on the list that once was
in my before- behind that fence segregating
then and now, that tower of bricks
of my stroke.

Now, my bucket list hangs on regaining whatever
sensation I can on my right side,
of walking on grass or sand and
holding my mother's hand in my now insensate right one
   and feeling the fine grains
or painless spikes of green roll below my right foot-
that currently dumb and unfeeling
part of me that once gulped down reality by the stride,
   that could once

converse with Earth and listen to the fable of its
  geography,
gathering up knowledge about its contact with our planet,
about gravity, about movement –
a currency I once endowed with devout passion.

Now,
my unstable,
stuttering gait
terrorizes me,
stoking intense electric agony down my
left leg, offering no
positional awareness to my right foot.

I long
to feel pressure,
to feel touch,
to feel something,
anything.

I long to taste food on the right side of
my mouth,
to feel my mother's embrace across my
spine on my right shoulder,
to type these words as opposed
to dictate them.

There is so much fear,
a choking noose about my neck,
and not knowing what is to come.

And yet, there is also immense beatitude—
a strange and ironic

cocktail of feeling cursed and blessed simultaneously.

Against predictions of doctors,
I survived a medical mishap that should have been
    otherwise.

It could have been otherwise.

It could have eradicated my breath.

No one knows what may happen next.

No physician nor roadmap can guide me on this zip-line.

I am the conductor of my body's disharmonious
orchestra, attempting to synthesize mellifluous music out
    of the entropy of being.

I am not sure who I am or who I can become.

All I can know is the resolve to become someone I want to
    be-
someone less afraid,
someone continually persistent, someone enlivened by
    the here and now-
by the happenings that dial me into and define me in this
adrift present until the future finds me in this
vulnerable darkness.

Ghost stories

I am haunted by my former self,
a respiring vestige I was and now carry,
a miscarriage of self-contained within
paper walls of wounded flesh.

There is a ghost wandering narrow pathways pervading
   my soul,
a human I called myself sequestered in shadowy purgatory
   of before
dithering between the once possible and the now
   implausible.

It feels as though there is a dead bird enshrouded within,
something yearning for flight that once flew across
   oceans,
but no longer is at all.

I attempt to find new ground-
to uncover a solid surface beneath feet,
one of which I can no longer feel,
to locate refuge, home, safety I never before
considered until I was breached of security,
neared the ledge of a final breath in this world-
unlaced and seamless,
unfinished and incoherent.

The recollections of my soul that once
harvested gallons of beauty and meaning have begun to
   fade away,
a bright turquoise bleeding into ever fainter hues until
   unsullied whiteness prevails.

But certain memories stick out, luminous candles in the
   dark-
my parents' tear-drenched faces forever
unready to countenance their daughter's proximity to
   death,
the spinal cord stroke searing their

27-year-old girl's brainstem,
desecrating the life she built out of untampered grit
she deemed impenetrable by the unthinkable to conceive
    or to prevent,
bifurcating her world into a before and after-
a Rubicon she could never cross as the once effusive
    circulation
between her and the universe,
a cord cut,
an unbearable breach,
a steep and unfathomable aggregate of loss collecting at
    the
base of their child's throat,
rendering swallowing and breathing heroic acts.

Just being became synonymous with defiant courage.

Existence morphed from a subconscious given into full-
    time occupation.

That beaming laboratory scientist
peering into a half dozen novels vanished-
their daughter replete with the desire to plumb depths of
    the
known and knowable
gone in a fraction of a second,
replaced by someone she does not yet,
or perhaps refuses to, adopt as herself.

But she has learned more, too much,
in the past 16 months
than in the sum total of her 28 years prior
and wishes the world could acquire her insight without

her plight and pillage.

She craves to become as paradoxically patient and
   unyielding as a river-
forever rushing away and forever returning home,
eternal dynamism
clasped within awesome stillness.

She has realized that neither simple nor complex
mathematics can formulate or integrate this life,
that being human inexorably entails having your
heartbroken a million times and mustering the
outrageous might to begin at the beginning,
that everything simply happens to us and
our one excruciating and astonishing task
is to be with that happening,
that anything can break us wide open-
splicing us into ever smaller fragments,
shards of shells we must collage again to fate's exponent-
not into the identical whole conches they once were
but into newfangled and, until then, unexplored
   adaptations of
togetherness, however messy,
however ineptly constructed.

Perfection perfectly skips over the point-
the art of wresting something never before
imagined out of contused fragility as reality
impales us, lashing out in thunderclaps that we are
   eternally ephemeral-
this flesh and bone brittle and breakable,
this Earth a living entity in which we are but for a finite
   ribbon

of time between soil and stars,
sparkling souls remarkably beautiful and mortal,
our lives forever incomplete and incompletable.

Ordinary note

When I find myself, a rare occurrence these days, it is not in the sloshing slurry of syllables, not in the overcast and overbearing downpour of words, but rather in the elegant spaces between them—in the reprieve, in the pause, in the purposeful lost artistry of being without doing, of thinking of nothing save for my breath flowing into and out of my torso, lending me novelty in each precious precarious moment.

This moment is all we will ever have.

I have learned that oftentimes, language hits a stumbling block against impenetrable trauma. You cannot delineate or define it for anyone outside of the circle to which it occurs; you cannot even find the words to approximate it for those undergoing it. We need an unimagined lexicon for this shadow-sphere in which we are simultaneously homeward bound and losing our way.

It simply is—

happenstance happening.

So, instead of exhausting Miriam Webster's anthology, I resort to lacunas, to margins and feeling marginalized by language and its holding power and by the world rushing by me on their cell phones leading normal lives, uttering mundane sentences, jotting down routine errands and assignments.

Oh, how many blessings drench and dazzle humanity

that transpire under the radar of registered attention.

Please take note.

Please permit the poise of unstructured silence to intervene,

to interject itself amidst the blurred hurry of schedules.

The cosmos is not reducible to a single variable.

There is no need, no way, to calculate through the brambles of being human.

They tell you that jealousy only hurts you. They tell you that anger and hostility only defile your spirit. They tell you that hatred only offends the hater, but it is impossible to at once be human inside a body with a beating heart and to not feel such emotions crest and drop like unending ocean when you have been hit at age 28 by the hammer of an unanchoring stroke—a fragile, invisible shoelace you forgot to double knot. I am not sure who the undefinable hoard of "they" references, or if that is of pertinent concern.

Tell me how to describe the ineffable, to define yourself and your trauma in the form of a narrative you can tell others when you are the first of your kind to outlive such a catastrophe.

You are the precedent, and who is there to guide you?

And the problem with trauma is that it cannot be contained, put into slumber like an anesthetized caged tiger. It is ineffable. It has no boundary. It does not even seem to have a through-line linking your tenses. It is simply here, monolithic and cruel, sitting with daggers in eyes in the pit of your throat, a plum pit you cannot swallow, nor will ever be able to swallow.

It seems I have crossed the line from bilateral Homo sapiens to half breed, to something half human, to something half here, a lingering once upon a lifetime ago luminary. But after all of the explaining, the story I attempted to carve out of my fiasco over the last year, I live within the open arms of serene beauty, of divine grace, of bliss, of presence in the absences, in the spaces between the words I will never have.

Fugitive

I awoke as someone else melting into science fiction,
burgeoning the distance between me and myself—
the person I was high on becoming.

A Picasso painting,
fugitive pieces of my elemental ecology
jolted out of alignment.

No segment of my life is where it ought to be.

My vision swirls into a cryptic kaleidoscope.

Nothing is nailed in its rightful place.

Screws stumble out of order.

Even the vase on the table is restless, resisting stillness.

All roves in an upside-down pendulum that hastens as the
    day drains hours.

My hearing dissolved on the right side of my cranium.

Taste limped from my right mouth.

I feel empty, save for the queasy grace of nerve pain, on
   my right body.

I am half here, half not.
I am present.
I disintegrate,
a bubble popping into thin air.

Strangers in the airport inspect me stationed in my
   wheelchair
like an exhibit in a museum,
an incommunicable affliction,
an out-of-order human on display,
a spider clawing on an unstable surface of the world,
a curiosity at arm's length,
a phenomenon behind dense, impenetrable glass—
my othership a predicament that could never befall them.

I am severed straight down my axis of symmetry.

Even the thoughts inside my brain are garbled, scrambled,
lubricated with lidocaine that prevents slippery
plots from adding up into novels—
a frictionless sense of free-fall of consciousness that
   threatens
my bibliophilic tendencies.

Who I am if not a devourer of fiction?

The harassed wires of my central nervous system are at a
   standstill that does not budge.

Even this very breath is premeditated.

These choppy words bluntly cut.

I am battling to retrain my bowels to migrate
    unidirectionally,
to relocate ribs I do feel dislocate,
to align a body off-kilter.

All of my reserves,
the totality of my energy, the grand sum of my troops,
the nerve fibers yet intact within my punctured brain,
and the vestiges of my vision, funnel into my urge to
mutate what is currently
surviving into one day thriving- however scarred and
    piecemeal.

I itch to sculpt a life out of these ashes.

I am disillusioned.

In this divorce from discomfort,
I bide time in undergrowth,
educating myself how to know nothing,
how to commence from scratch.

I yearn to wake into wonder.

Breadcrumbs

I am petrified of what I can no longer feel, what I can no longer
perceive, what I can no longer spiral into proof out of words, a linguistic mathematics—once a steel bastion of givens that added
up, now a faraway sleight of hand, Lego pieces in my brain. There
is a rush of mayhem now, an onslaught of catastrophic disaster
and despair that digs a hole in the armamentarium of my spirit.

Everything has splintered, fractured into billions of pieces I will never collect, a glass figurine that can never be restored. It seems I lose myself each day, as I endeavor to locate the outline of my absent right side. I have forgotten all I seek to remember and recall all I seek to forget. I am vanquished of imprints on the right side of my spinal cord: a flicker of wind, my mother's caress, my father's clean-shaven cheek, dripping tap water, the feeling of my hands encircling a mug, blazing summer heat sinking its way into my skin.

Yet the trauma dawdles, a blaring stab of recollection. I remember verbatim, as though it were a tragic play; that morning I awoke from a routine cervical procedure and was slammed into the afflicted side of the galaxy—the inverted edge of my existence—as I groped for my right side and screamed when I could not find it, when my brain could not detect it in space, when my defective radar deflected in the dark alone pen of disarming disability, left with but my left side.

And I recall my childhood innocence, its breezy carryover into college. I see this girl who is not me, but is me, in her starkly blue oversized winter coat, as if I were looking through the looking glass at both a stranger and myself. I have become unfamiliar within native skin. The trappings often deceive me into the delusion that I am still here, that my right side is alright, even though I cannot perceive it in the slightest, even though I have lost control of my entire life at age 28, even though the nightmare of my reality filled with a torrent of overwhelm from which I must disengage and disappear.

The aftershock of my spinal cord stroke is still shocking, has yet to be metabolized, has yet to settle within the cavern of my spirit that is both broken and unyielding. There is a part of me that is lost. There is a part of me I am still working on finding a path back towards, or at least a foot-trail of distant breadcrumbs that may point me in the approximate direction of whom I may become within the shackles of the nervous system unhinged by a trauma so perplexing that even medical experts are flabbergasted.

> I miss all of the things that once came naturally,
> that once never felt like things I could miss.
> All I long for is everything
> I never knew I had before,
> and I vow that I will never forget
> whatever I can recover from this
> undertow of loss.

If there is a God, or any taskmaster orchestrating skies and destinies, I beseech you to just give me back sensation in one limb, one digit, on my right side. Anything will suffice.

> These bites of poem—
> this life in the preserve of words—
> is the only variety I possess.

So, I will write my way all the way to right margin, scuttling the pen in my vocal cords to carry me on its back wherever I can go, even if my right half is irretrievable from the throttling tug of disability.

Palimpsest

The penciled past ghosted, written over by the
    unforeseeable present-
a tongue tripper, a mind bender, a soul somersaulting
    through tortuous truths.

The prison of disability is a river overflowing with memory-
a stirring of sadness at being forgotten,
at becoming emblematic of a bad omen in your eyes,
at being the one who vividly recalls the life entombed,
    extinguished-
a wondrously bold and majestic sunset washed into
    blackness,
into a profusion of overcast winter nights.

We are all mortal wrapped in shells of time.

Maybe the stars remember my name, my past that was
    never granted the opportunity to catch up with my
    present.

Maybe I am the stardust I always was- this terrifically
    terrible creature of finitude-
my potential a secret secluded between me and the silken
    sky.

The horrific gift of being overwritten, oftentimes, against
    our wills.

That searcher of the known world once so part and parcel
    of my being
has not endured alongside my remarkable yet asymmetric
    physical form miffed by my too young stroke.

An aching and excruciating pain of being in a body that
  cracks, a divestiture, an unexpected and exasperating
  transgression exactly when I was allegedly in a
  physician's healing hands.

And it has only taken me roughly three decades and this
  brutal confrontation with reality to realize that the only
  underground aspect of this life I know keenly is the
  unknown.

The unknown is my mother.

The unknown is the seed of my becoming, which
  will ignite the flame of being anew if I afford myself
  permission to emerge into a pattern sewn together we
  can never stitch of our own accord nor recognize before
  the sweeping fabric suddenly appears.

Wordless loss and tumultuous trauma tell you in
emboldened letters that this world is packed with a
  privation of knowable controls-
that we must let go of this ostensibly human famine of
  intellect, even if this means relinquishing our grips on
  the reigns of ourselves-
our pasts, presents and futures-
that we will all die so many times in this singular life,
cultivate parades of palimpsests until our breaths trail off
and we merge, once and for all, with the crucible of
  darkness,
expansive silence and intermittent starlight, atomizing into
  the subliminal yet sublime cosmology of the unknown,
  unconquerable textiles of existence.

No harbinger

In single breath, this frail Earth may buckle beneath your
  feet,
plunging you into the undefined discomfiture of doubt,
dismantling you ad hoc into the sidelined swollen
  crumbling
justice of the world you mistook for fortified truth.

But being human comes at the cost of our own breaking,
our own disappointed disappearance,
being wounded to such a degree that we must forge a
frighteningly unfamiliar frontier.

I feel like something disposable,
a paper airplane,
falling through a crack
in nature.

I nosedive and descend.

This falling has no floor.

I continue to tumble downwards
into the padlock chains of disability,
forced to interpret
a new pattern of existence,
to reshape my undone self that I project
onto the unknown face of the universe,
to emancipate myself from the
grinding gridlock of
devastation.

This world has broken

my heart wide open,
has severed my mind
a million times over.

Against this strange edge,
in which I am alive but not fully living,
my inner mathematician has come to the
petrifying conclusion
that there is
no arithmetic,
no algorithm,
no accounting,
for the things we do,
for the things done to us.
Before will always be better.

For 15 months in the after of my ruination,
I resented my body for deserting me-
for forgetting how to process sensation,
for its ineptness to repair me,
to seal over the looming canyon in my world so
I could once again stand and feel my own feet.

My anger soared,
a bird casting its wings skyward,
at my body's retaliation.

But I must grant myself absolution.

For since this brainstem stroke,
my body has soldiered valiantly to breathe.

I can only pray that it will always
be hungry for the words,

my one lulling source of fuel.

For if they leave, what residue resides?

I have forgotten how to converse with hope.

Maybe I can practice the placebo of belief-
compel my distraught mind
to mine shafts of light in this darkness,
to find grounding in this fraught quiet,
to sense lightness pour through
my physical body once again.

I want to gather up more of me,
oh, so very much more.

Tears are filling up the well of my breaking.

Does mourning ever wither in this lifetime?

How can I begrudge a body
endeavoring so ardently to survive that asks
for so little in return?

The evidence of my survival is
deflating,
defeating,
deafening,
an enduring tattoo of my own mortality
that renders this moment penetratingly,
painfully present,
its inflection point
too narrow and steep.

I yearn for the mundane

to become more mundane.

This wheelchair that replaces my legs.

That commode that lingers by my bedside.

The oxygen concentrator in the corner of my bedroom.

This walker conjoined to my being to carry me short
  distances.

This terribly, beautifully broken body is
composed of such soft fabric—
flesh crocheted together by tears,
absurdly buoyant laughter quaking through my living
  nightmare,
my mother's hand between my shoulder blades,
the eruption of restless silences in lieu of feelings
untouchable and unreachable by speech,
an enduring soul that defies it all
to be with these fissures
that not even time can heal.

In coming unmade
from the pivot point of all the
threads that yoked me to the world,
I have learned that the finish line of existence
I once raced towards as a given for nearly three decades
does not, in fact, exist at all, nor does the race itself-
that the future forever retreats no matter how close
we presume we come to its crossing,
that enough is never quite enough,
that being human means never being sated,
that we live unfinished lives no matter how

fortune randomly plays for or against us,
that, in the end, all we really want is to
see and to be seen
in all of our fractured luminosity,
to need and to be needed,
to explore the world and,
at our end,
to exclaim,
"I was here, witnessed and bore witness."

But the disabled, like me, engage in a
ruthless battle of hide and seek with themselves and the
    world,
are paradoxically the lonely few who acknowledge
this truth and yet fail to realize it,
because for us this beatific world of wild gambling
is one in which we are only invited to observe from afar,
not to engage to the extent of our innermost desires
we aspire to keep secreted in our bones for fear
of coming more undone than we already are.

Glitches

The heartbreaking truth is beautiful—
the journey is always from the known to the unknown,
from where the land ends to where something might
    begin.

It may be a drowning sea.

It may be a desolate desert.

The uncertainty is petrifying,

a jogging jolt of electricity
rinsing across axons.

Right side,
we officially need counseling over this jarred
spinal cord but may be too far removed from
each other to view the problem properly at this juncture-
too adrift from each other's reception
across your noncommittal synapses,
my choppy nervous system.

There is no guidebook for how to do this—
how to divorce or to remarry
your bisected corporality.

We are transactional now.

For, not even our once upon a time
iteration of romance at the bone of us
can be recovered in memory,
a wound sealed
tightly over by scarred skin.

We are but footnotes in each other's biographies.

You have been surgically excised from my life,
replaced with surplus shame-
my body a shine of secrets kept,
its fracture lines cemented over.

Are you in the alternate universe of that almost adjacent
    life?

Where is that version of us?

I am not quite beside myself.

I am, you are, elsewhere.
I am someone else without you,
without everything we nearly should have had.

There is no user interface,
no interference mechanism,
for this sort of malware,
this malady of a penetrated nervous system.

Reader, I recognize that this story is
anything but reassuring or steadying,
but it is candidly me:
pain-stained and asymmetric but true,
oh so very brutally true.

This is my, our, story.

It has me in its clutches,
but I must tell it,
to let the words rattle air
because that it is the extent of my authority now:
to bear up all of the secrets I can no longer keep at bay.

Here they are.

I am giving them to you.

I am going somewhere—
traveling beyond the shackles of my body,
beyond the manacles of tragedy,
beyond anything I could ever
think to get beyond.

Because here I am.

Here this very sentence is.

Here is something broken,
perhaps irreparably,
but not without hope,
not without faith,
not without wings that carry me
elsewhere on the seam of imagination.

If only I were a bird.

If only life complied with my if-onlys.

But the universe does not care.

The universe stomps its foot on me over and again,
a shoe slamming against cosmic breaks,
but I continue to find grounding
on the path of possibility.

Because along this untraveled,
unmapped terrain,
a paratrooper persists,
a scientist hunches,
a mother gives birth to a healthy daughter,
an average 28-year-old is married,
an unadulterated innocence percolates,
and anything can happen.

I can happen.

I do not have a cervical cord or a brainstem injury.

I can become anything.

So can you.

I can transgress the thick red tape of disability
and become the woman
I always sought to become.

The universe and its callous entropy cannot stop me from
    defining myself.

Although this path of possibility narrows by the day,
I can still swerve along it for a while and
become the designer of my fate,
if you believe fate exits.

And who cares about definitions
that will always be ill-equipped to contain us,
if I can string words together into an
instrument that allows my soul to sing a little,
and occasionally confers
order out of ruthless circumstance?

I refuse to starve myself of joy any longer,
to prevent its glistening beads from
indenting novel neural networks
I can skim even as I wrestle my trauma.

Here I go—
hatching a sunrise out of this wintering,
dripping my tears onto the
safe negative space
of this page,
lubricating the binary finitude of the alphabet
with the infinite spectrum of emotion.

Let us be here—
at the impossibility immersive and immense

spaces between words,
between each other-
malleable connective tissue
of metaphor.

Because in the end,
we are all just practicing the art of being broken,
doggedly seeking to emerge whole along some
path of possibility that may lead anywhere.

Conclusion

The speaker's footing in language and her return to scientific terminology intensifies, as does her audacity to look into her rearview mirror to examine her condition and life with both clarity and levity. She evolves in step with her poetics and focuses on drawing courage to move forward in spite of her unremitting disability.

Movement IV
Hall of mirrors

Introduction

The speaker's poems are both reflecting and refracting across time, and in this section, they are beginning to metamorphose as meditations on the mortal pendulum, the body's adaptability, its inevitable decay, and her parents' sustaining shelter. She catalyzes her passion for math and science into a poetics of self-reclamation as she rewrites calculus and discovers ways to incorporate a new math and science into her poetry.

Moments of oxygen

I am awestruck by each tree—
its commitment to posture,
a perfect spinal cord, if nature ever perfected anything,
its lodging firmly underfoot while reaching
with slender and impossibly long arms
towards the crystalline firmament,
no matter how inclement the weather.

The tree motivates me
to unkink my spinal cord
from the stronghold of trauma,

from acquiescence to the inadequacy
swiping through my mind—
a voice to which my physical body
replies by arcing ever more inwards
as though I must contort myself into something
implausibly microscopic,
as though I were incompetent
to still call myself a member of the human race,
as though I were ducking for cover beneath a mighty
    wave
or preparing for a raging riptide of flames.

I marvel at the covert cryptography, the wordless and
    tuneless
musical exchange between roots,
generating fellowship out of sonorous silence,
a palpable quiet we could perhaps hear
if only we took the time,
the tabooed leisure,
to listen to muffled voices to which
we have grown allergic in our repressive arrogance.

My undoing bequeathed me with time to hear the
    inaudible.

I throb to grasp the grammar of the arboreal tongue,
to knock on the doors of the trees' sentences,
to trace the shape of their wordless vocabulary.

For my injury has installed within me the truth that even
    the emptiest
forms of silence take on certain
convexity or concavity,

a different type of fullness demanding an orphaned form
  of intimate listening.

My disability inches me nearer to this sensitivity,
to seat myself in faith in that tree beckoning just beyond
  my window.

And, while my world often feels death-drenched,
I remain fastidiously curious about that willow's experience
  of articulation outward
from its solid and stoic center,
its growth in the nest of immobility,
its weaving of itself towards sunlight, however faint,
however muted behind curtains of clouds.

In the quaking wake of
unspeakable loss of my body and of my existence
as I fathomed my coordinates in the here and now,
there is a profusion of tears—
perhaps sufficient in quantity to water an entire forest.

I have come to worship
every wren,
every shrub,
every lily in a field beyond my field of view,
each blade of grass I can but see within my internal
  circuitry,
and every developing and decaying entity
that musters the acrobatic intrepidity
to cultivate itself as it unabashedly engages with its own
  death.

I never before acknowledged the pumping autonomic
  astonishing cycles of nature,

the rises and falls that make and unmake us all at once.

So, in the company of the tree beyond my window,
I will continue to donate to and to receive from the
    recycling atmosphere.

I will continue to be embodied carbon,
a collage of atoms colliding into selfhood as I fight for life,
stretching through space and time
towards the light, however wan and far off,
however cruel and mercurial this rapid-fire existence,
however adjacent death,
however tattered my physicality,
because right here,
I find moments of oxygen on the ocean floor, a
    magnificent and munificent
hatching of a non-native self as I converse with instants of
    breakthrough,
the wondrously transient nature of nature.

I am finally invited back to rest in my body,
into the gift of presence, these sacred bleeding Ten
    Commandments
of being human.

Wrinkles in the dialogue

My consciousness, unlike my external life, which only adopts the blistering shade of disability, is a split-screen. All too often fraught in paresthesia—intractable and misguided nerve impulses my right side sends to what remains of my central nervous system—like letters mailed to the wrong address, and in the muck of vestibular symptoms that leave me in a heady vertiginous delusion of rocking back-and-forth across space, I prey on ephemera of normalcy. A Taylor Swift song enters my left eardrum, and suddenly, I am plunged backwards in time, no longer a broken 28-year-old, a reject ejected from what was once a blessed life. Or I engage in a conversation with a friend; we discuss a book on trauma, and rapidly, I am excerpted out of my own hardship, viewing it as a science from the outside, rather than dwelling within its firm grip—my body and brain no longer keeping the scarred score of my militance against disaster.

At the juncture at which life seemed to confer answers, to parse a path towards a PhD and relationships, the very questions themselves drastically changed. The ground beneath me not only shifted but also shattered. I devastatingly fell beneath myself. I am not a religious person, nor was I ever, but I would not call myself areligious nor secular. I could designate myself spiritual. I could pen myself into some category of faith, if classifications mattered. My heritage is Jewish, and thus I am a Jew, regardless of the labels I choose to wear. But I refuse to believe in a God who keeps a record, in a Devine who inscribes people in the book of life or death, in an Almighty reachable through a direct fulfillment of commandments, as though actions added up that way, in a God who keeps score, as though life were one protracted football game. I do not feel that God struck me down nor that God permitted me to continue respiring, despite the stroke to my medulla that should have, that could have, demarcated this very sentence beyond the purview of possibility.

Everything happens. And there is no rational backbone, no reason, no sacred secret behind the veil of circumstance, no shadow or undercurrent that molds one human to handle suffering more adequately than another. I will leverage my fleeting respites from my concussion and trauma as they emerge—tiny seashell fragments, sacrosanct wrinkles in the dialogue—as if I were welcoming the most sought-after and unannounced visitors into my arms. This is because the infinite now is whispering into my ear that I contain more than finite flesh vanquished of all feeling on the right side, depleted of the desire for food and drink, deprived of depth perception, and so many other symptoms and ruthless side-effects of a tragedy so beleaguering that it has transfigured the topography of my entire life.

At this point, I will take whatever life proffers, because one day, a soul will reach out and want to gently touch mine, will need to touch mine through riptides of grief, and I will let them know that I have genuinely been there, that I can gracefully chart their journey upwards towards the sun, that you can rest in dissonance with me, our fingers interdigitated.

Pendulum

Trace it back to mathematical precision, to calculable
    amplitudes of bobs swinging from pivot points
    migrating through equilibriums,
to the brisk pulse of physics,
to the Han Dynasty's seismometer,
to Galileo Galilei, to the pendulum clock stuttering
    through time,
to the indeterminate throbbing masses of our spirits
    oscillating
between fear and faith,

erosion and emergence,
pain and purpose.

Bodies incline into the beyond,
arching towards the horizon,
bowed, indirect, unstable-
my limbs readily dispatching themselves
from their sockets by my connective tissue disease.

Remind me, what do ordinary days taste like?

Are Monday and Tuesday coated with the same flavoring?

Pendulum—
I am the process.

A necessary nail in my universe popped out of its groove,
apocalyptically thrusting me out of the nexus of my next
    moment,
the bomb of my being detonated while I was tranquilized
    by anesthesia, caught in the dreamcatcher of my youth,
    of once upon a time, and then, a flip of a switch-
the raging, deafening, roaring, impossible, resounding
silent alarm of pain splintering through my body,
untouchable by words,
a wound ripping its way through me—
the blazing flames in my right scalp, the catatonia of my
right hemisphere draining feeling, nerve pain that now
    jogs, a tripwire combusting
electricity in every direction—
across my pelvis,
down the inseam of my left leg,
up my head and into my jaw—

hibernating me into claustrophobia of self,
unbearable, unbelievable.

I am the journey.

I am my own end.

My survival against the odds—
too outsized, too overcast, thoughts surrounding
it so heavy they must be put down before my arms detach
    from my torso in this after,
distancing me from everything—
from schedules,
calendars,
friends,
family,
the future that once felt as perceptible as the present.

Pendulum—
from the deserted desert of disability,
these pithy stanzas—
a postcard, billowing smoke, an arm extending its way
    across oceans to you.

I reside light years away from everything I once took to
    be true and real, even from words, as they exude and
    express their way up through my throat, legible volumes
    of verbal vomit of the soul- for no vocabulary can
    contain rivers of sadness,
a maelstrom that feels like it is strangling me from within
    as I grieve my own loss of self, the memories slowly
    slipping away, my right side with them.

My entire galaxy blinks in the blackest bruise of the sky.

But words are all I have left.

So let us be here together with what remains and be
grateful for what is so beautiful in this broken world.

Oh, how we mortal creatures vacillate between the
    excruciating
and the magnificent.

A pinprick of awareness—the electrocution within as my
    right ribs
successfully break free from their sockets—
the blistering dissonance of feeling, an air raid of my core,
the juncture between my brain and my right half
nonexistent, a picture fading out of itself.

This homing missile, a wall of needles on which I hang
    internally,
sharpens one sensation at the cost of all others,
placing earplugs in my ears, masking my eyes.

I am held in the captivity of white noise,
silent darkness, bottomless, penetrating pain.

And then the sun rises,
and through the dart of pain, something effortlessly
majestic emerges in being alive in the instant of dawn
    when colors begin to break free out of the depths of
    swallowing dark,
the morning cracking into a new day,
slamming into me with both horror and amazement of
being this beating heart, this fractured flesh.

We can make meaning out of the formlessness of
    circumstances that you cannot change but that can
    change you, if you let them.

Helix of self dissipates, that Elly I loved trapped in ember,
outside of time, liminal, eternal, on the see-saw of the
        pendulum
of self, her outline shimmering with innocence-
the uninterrupted flow of breath, unperturbed instincts
anchored in the brainstem that forgot me in this after.

Oh, brain, once so tactfully eager to resolve complex
    algebra problems
without pen and paper,
please recall my being-
the once even orchestra of breath,
    hunger, thirst- blessed empty feelings I could once fill.

In the unpaved, winding weeds of trauma, you see no
    footpath, no blueprint.

Your body, the only roadmap in sight, is where you land,
    without a native tongue, without a compass, a bind
    survivor of the dark.

Pendulum—
bless this soul as still embraces letters, even after her own
narrative twisted its neck on her.

Pendulum—
networks of neurons circumnavigating my spine, fraught
    in a riptide of flames,
without respite, without a fire squad to douse this agony.

This poem is writing itself,

as I lean into the pen of my vocal cords,
as I lean into everything now,
denting my way into the universe,
my right side mopped clean by
my stroke of sensation.

My right half, now an excavation site of memory I thumb
    through,
a flip book, this wasteland of self-
that tartan jumper writing the world into comprehension
    in math classrooms,
calculating amplitudes of pendulums in Physics textbooks,
analyzing her way through The Wasteland
she thought only bled through parchment, not virgin skin.

She was always a fractal shy, a Fibonacci number away,
    from wiring her cosmos into completion, a sheet ironed,
    a Band-Aid on the open wound of the world,
holding her together.

Pendulum—
an echo crescendos through the walls of recollection
in the Holland tunnel of my concussed body.

The dial tone into my before-
the permanency of things seemed to press her into herself,
a seatbelt against tribulations, against her suddenly
    metamorphosing into the protagonist in Kafka's *The Trial*.

She thought she could study her way, head sleeping on
    open books,
through trauma, out of the forbidding

socket of pain, out of being human, out of the fragility she
    knew as an intellectual project, not as a framework for
    existence.

Suddenly, the rubric reversed on her—
she became
The Trial,
The Wasteland,
A Separate Piece,
Darkness at Noon—
unimaginable realities stored in novels, too unreal for the
    reality of mortality.

Oh,
these books turned their backs on me,
reach their way, parchment crossing the threshold of skin,
into the shuddering essence of my emergence.

Now these words floating on the page feel like the parts
    of her body- so broken, so inadequate in their own
    lonesomeness, dependent like this now rendition of self
on walkers,
on wheelchairs,
on oxygen concentrators,
on portable commodes,
on this uncharted,
unchoreographed,
under-appreciated white canvas
on which I slowly drip the paint of words—
azure and violet of my soul,
incandescence in darkness.

This is where the light grows.

Pendulum—
I am my own masterpiece.

I know these verses come at the expense of finding and
losing myself over and again, as I learn the grace
hiding within my body's breaking, unlearn all of
the knowledge that never made me as intact within as my
  physical breaking did.

Pendulum—
I am lost.

Pendulum—
I am whole.

Pendulum—
I am.

Pendulum—
I am a stray cat within the alley of disability.

But I am roaming through windows of these words,
etching the outer boundary of my shadow,
dancing between what we must forsake and the light we
  can
always locate, if we grant ourselves the courage to find it.

In this dark cavern of self, I am undefinable—
student no longer,
scientist unmade,
a body besieged, but a soul
that still sings and sings.

This is my anthem.

Come join me.

Art project

I am living fragments of a body in aftershocks,
which falters to define me but permits me to redefine life,
   to make myself anew.
An avalanche rebounds within my chest as I stutter these
   words,
stimulating orchestral beauty out of Stravinsky discord-
the abused child of uncertainty and disaster.

I am atomic- my life continually pixelating before my eyes,
the future I compiled with undo diligence
but a castle built of sand exposed to a riptide.

I was once so much more than a medical enigma,
a roiling tumble of trauma.

I will not renounce my past.
I will not even aim fruitlessly to make sense of my injury, of
   my life,
of the parts of my soul that feel strewn across the floor and
   on
the verge of being swept under the rug.
I will take all these shards of glass and make something of
   them.

I will not delude myself into redirecting my way towards
   the future
I intended, but I will navigate towards beginning again,
   towards a refusal to give into the pain that seeps into my
   body, towards being gentler, supple, tender with
myself as if I were someone else I yearn to love.

This trauma will be my tree trunk, and I will learn to sprout
   branches.
I am so decomposed at this point that even quantum
   physicists
would be at a standstill to tape the vestiges of my spirit
   back together.
Perhaps this tangent is irrelevant if these intellectuals do
   not invest in the spiritual realm.
But that is besides my point, if I have one at all.

Must I?
Do you always need a pivot to hold onto as a thought
   filters through your psyche?

Because of this, I can check one fear off of my long tally of
   fears.
I no longer fear being broken, being asunder.
And out of my remains, I will grow myself anew.
I will build myself out of these ashes into more than a
   survivor,
into a tendon of my own strength.
This trauma is educating me how to reconfigure my soul-
   that is my art project.

Pass me the scissors, cardboard, and glitter.
Let us begin being shiny put-together beings we redeem.

Confluence

Memories have become slippery things by now, a fading whirl
of images that desaturate with time. Life is slackening my once
durable hold on my former self: her scent, flashes of electricity in
her smile, the glistening turquoise of her eyes. I peer at images of

myself, hesitantly daring to look over my own shoulder, at stages of development—observing myself at age 3 in a jean jumper, blonde ringlets wilting in the humid wind or another or me walking at the dawn of college hand-in-hand with a friend down the winding Concord Avenue. I question how much more distance reality will splice between me and my former self, between me and the woman I strove to embody. It seems like a physics problem in which the velocity and acceleration unwittingly accrue on me, widening the space between me and myself, between my before and my now, between what could-have-been and what is.

The alleyway has grown immeasurably vast and is now a boulevard I can no longer cross, even through the lens of memory, which is sliding into pixelated fog. There is no anger in this self-annihilation. There is only the touch and go of sadness and fear of how much more I can vanish from myself. I look at, and abruptly look away from, these still-lives of the person I once was without malice, but with the meek interest of an observer witnessing a flipbook featuring someone I once knew, perhaps even cherished.

I am pioneering the brutal art of surviving the day, which is proving not so simple, which is proving more complex a problem than anything I solved in quantum physics classrooms. There is no spare time to reconfigure the splinters of my soul into a configuration appropriate for my transgressed body, put through the crosshatching rings of fire of a stroke.

I am uncertain how much faith resides within my bank account of self.

I am uncertain what I can assemble out of my remains.
The land on which I once stood has smoldered,
without warning,
into a lopsided
precipice.

Hang onto the landslide,
the confluence of then and now,
with me.

Do not risk letting go.

The drop is more dramatic
than you know.

It always is.

That is why we must submerge
ourselves in the present.

Even though that which I seek is elusive, I refuse to
    surrender to the mountains of terror, to the loud
    pierce of pain buried so deep I cannot even reach it, to
    everything that immerses me in too much feeling and to
    everything that is no longer in contact with my nervous
    system.

All I can do is be within the parameters of now.
All I can do is attempt to acquiesce to someone in me I no
    longer fear.
All I can do is marshal enough grit to soften into feeling
less segmented,
a tad more complete,
a bit less charred,

a fraction more hopeful,
a sliver more expansive,
rehearse patience with patience,
whatever definitions those words
now adopt into their fluctuating spines.

I reached bottom—
sunk beneath the undertow of grueling
circumstance that defies language's capacitance—
but there is a narrow shaft of light
within the ashes of my spirit
yet kicking upward.

So, I—
a gardener of luminosity—
will tend to it with flickering courage
to flex the musculature of light,
so it's now uneven pulse emulsifies
into measured visual,
glowing music,
a portrait of endurance.

Endurability

As a year transpires since my stroke,
I glean the critical distinction between resilience and
    endurability—
between the buoyancy of return and
the defiant audacity to fight against adversity
caged within my own skin.

I am forbidden from slipping under the barrier into my
    before—

incapable of bouncing back,
into the kingdom of the well,
unauthorized to crack open the door,
or even a peephole,
into my past and
peer into it for a dash of a second,
to flood the well of recollection.

There is nothing to return to from right here:
this instant, this sentence, this undying sense of an ending.

When my connective tissue disease posed my primary
    conundrums,
not this lean adjunct to suffering,
casting limbs out of alignment,
I slid shoulders into sockets,
racing to emigrate to the remedied before state.

The frisbee was passed back, a return key tapped, and I
    was restored to what was.

What a wonder.

But now, my undoing is final—irrevocable, incorrigible.

There is no button I can press, no spell you can hum to
    return me to my former blessed operating mode.

My task is now survival, and for that, endurance is the only
    critical ingredient.

There is a fraction in me whose numerator fluctuates,
calibrating my desire to yield to the persistent agony,
to the heft of my shadow and loss that gnaw at the
    marrow of my bones,

burrowing my skeleton until I feel too hollow to be real,
for this story to be mine.

Is it mine?

Is it yours?
Someone else, please volunteer to pick up the cudgel of
   this narrative,
if only temporarily, or, better yet, find a way to incinerate it,
so I can live inside the one preserved
in the kingdom of my resilience, of my before.

I am right against an edge.
I write against this precipice of palpitating disquiet-
inexpressible and indelible grief that presses hard
against the blunt implement of language and its inertia to
   contain the festering uncontainable.

For what motivates us to write if not some corner, some
   razor of being?

I am no longer the resilient one, smile bioluminescent
   through her before gentle shackles of sorrow so light she
   did not even register them.

I am now the young adult indispensably dependent on
   her parents to press her onwards, to enlarge her ability
   to endure so that she may do so for another day, another
   hour, another minute.

Inside of these words, inside of this bleeding and beating
   heart,
I muster resolve to seek self in sentences and permit
   language to encircle me,
to expand in my endurability so I may release myself

fleetingly from anxiety and distress as the rush of words
carry me in another direction towards
another world liberated of trauma.

Raw bones

I am kindred with the coverlet of blackness decorating predawn hours, as though the sky were preparing for Earth's funeral, uncoiling me from solitude, endowing me with fortitude to open my eyes to the bare fact of being alive inside a body in discordant distress. Be it three or four in the morning, the darkness is an invitation to locate a massive paintbrush and color myself in black acrylic, to merge into something united with nature. Arising to an absence of sensation on my right side—which now feels more like a presence as the weight of time compounded by grief accumulates—once caught me off-guard, an unanticipated punch in the stomach. However, now it adopts a faded accent of fear because I am not alone. I am one with the uncertain night as it trips its way into the early morning, caught, like me, in the liminal space between what is and what is not. There is no real way to define these early hours, just as I elude categories and definitions. The morning is when my mourning begins to fester, when the darkness gives way to light that sheds far too much brightness on just how torn asunder my reality has become. I am practicing how to be less petrified. I am practicing how to become like the tree bark over there or like the tulip in that bed, soaking in the raw bones of this moment, refining the art-form of being. I am trying to teach each of my cells to offload their immense baggage, to let go of the story of my pain. I am trying to become dynamically placid, to simultaneously become whatever the moment permits while being at peace with my own unbecoming. Although my world feels brutally closefisted and uninhabitable, I am trying to locate a small opening to let the light in. The darkness may be my ally. The night may be my confidant. Daybreak may break me. But I am learning how to remake myself in each moment, to become less scared of small splinters of light so that I can grow into something broken, but beautiful—a tree shorn of several branches following a storm, raw bones that gently hum.

Alchemy

I was once so filled to the brim with words, with syllables, diction, synonyms and antonyms, and a gush of letters hanging together into cogent diction. But now, language languishes, no longer coheres. The vocabulary collage is creased, inadequate to exude objective truth. Although we swing towards this notion, achieving its pure state is out of reach of human hands and human minds. Everything in this world shifts: even the constants that once defined your life, even the memories that you call your past, even the numbers pressed onto chalkboards.

Nothing summates like basic arithmetic. There are shades within monotone if you seek them. Math is beauty in its abstract incarnation but fails to exist, spine erect, inside the mundane flowing flux of days. It is up to us to make things add up, to multiply life by invested meaning, and to mold substance out of uncultured matter.

Even the words I once worshiped as a schoolgirl jumped and jumbled out of context in this addled brain post-stroke. Not only because my brain feels like something archaic yet newborn, something foreign, something transplanted from someone else's body, but because the words feel far less worthy of their ascent to the throne, to the regal and incredibly important heights they once scaled across my neurons.

> I am still simmering on constellations of memory,
> shoving scintillating starry clouds into imagination
> to let them mushroom there unhemmed.

I am not sure who I am, what I am, or what words can wrap around my now. I limp through the world on a left leg; my insensate right limb quests to cull its way home but is no longer fed the sensory sustenance it deserves.

> Medical care heedlessly and haphazardly
> bartered for malfeasance,
> landing me in the Dust Bowl of calamity,
> my spine forgetting to elicit fibers
> within my right interior,
> the once blessed unnoticed
> white noise of neurons firing
> lapsing into sober silence.

Yet there is a spirit that resists the resistance of the universe—the waves that crash against the unknown of my right side. I am still here. I am still learning what it means to be broken open, what it means, or what it once meant, to be whole.

> I am settling into my fugitive fragments.
> For what other occupation can I aspire?

For what else should I aim but to be OK with not being
  OK?
I am not sick with sorry for myself,
for the loss that has crippled and rippled
through my estranged being.

I am learning to live with unsettling uncertainty without being
unsettled, without fraying my exposed and vulnerable nervous
system. I am learning to live in perpetual fear without being petrified of the overwhelm ricocheting through my bereavement.

  I am bowing into the paradox at the beating center of
    being human.
  I am learning that at all costs.
  I am the cost.
  I am paying,
  even through insolvency.

The token of time will undress who I may become, how I might
architect myself into someone I long to be—someone who is
not a scientist, a mother, or an Olympian, but who is a pilgrim
in process, weeding out the darkness so it ultimately presents a
tapered stream of sunrise.

Womb

  Our first darkness unremembered, stale silence of our
    budding voices,
  the branding of inheritance, a belly button—
  my now invisible bridge once so tactile and seen between
    me and my mother,

our first schism as life cuts our umbilical cords, wrenches
  us out of known solace,
leaving us indiscriminately alone with ourselves.

Oh the perfidy of promises undelivered, now
  undeliverable.

Womb—
I ache to return to your familiar dark depths, to my
  mother's warm shelter.

Womb—
a possible crater between me and my mother no longer
  viable.

We begin where I end.

Womb—
I carved a new umbilical cord,
upending the sweep of evolution, out of staggering brutal
  suffering.

Womb—
a tunnel of light, knowing we kindle as our eyes converse
  the topography of our souls.

We are suspended from the world, immersed in the gravity
  of our own galaxy.

Womb—
we resume the conversation, picking up the threads of
  tapestry begun at my conception,
now on the far-off island of infirmity.

My stroke, our dial tone, my delete key that life pressed
  and pressed until my future expired.

We are but tendrils of smoke of flesh that merge with the
crucible of creation.

Do you know how breakable, how fleeting and penetrable
you are?

Womb—
a blockade against truculent truth, unspeakable, unspoken
silence of savage and harsh retaliations that sideline me,
reshape me.

Illuminate the road of this quest, the X-ray of my desolate
soul journeying to light, visited too often by gruesome
isolation and cries.

Womb—
let me be 28, just for a moment.

Let me at least dream of it as my soul undergoes
transformation, transportation, transcendence-
as I both reenter my mother's womb and my own womb,
learning to hear the muted small still voice within on
which existence hinges, which you never hear unless you
are banished into yourself by destabilizing catastrophe
that tears you out of your own life.

How searing the blade of my redaction.

Womb—
since age 27, I gorged on melancholy- on loss and death
in life.

But no more.

No more.

For here I am, freeing the trapped knowing, a bird so long
  constrained,
with the wrench and screw of suffering.

Womb—
part of me still pains to crawl back into my mother's
  yawning body.

I discern consciousness leaking out, dissonance and
  distance between me and the world-
the ravenous learner of information no longer.

Trauma made me asymmetric internally-
my right side dislodged from my brain, the vanishing half
  of me I no longer sense.

Womb—
this crater of feeling, letters exchanged between
  hemispheres of my body in foreign tongues.

I am a voyaging poem articulated in my injured spine.

Womb—
erasures abound more than answers in this word.

I am a respiring translocation, a living manuscript laced
  with lacunae.

Are you?

Womb—
no quantity of mechanistic comprehension of the body
  will peel away the pulse
of mystery at its innermost workings.

I will tend to this empty nest of my right side, fill the
   vacuum with a garden as I till fertile soil of this half of me
   suspended in animation.

I thirst to watch sun fall upon grass in each season of time.
For no light splinters the same way twice.
Each dance a new kindling, a new beginning.

Come join me as we observe the world spin.

Womb—
if only I could again be all skinned knees, tangled curls,
   arms dangling from monkey bars,
legs pumping the dynamo of atmosphere on swings.

But I am, you are, all of my palimpsests, all of my whole
   breaking, right here in these words, as plain as blood
   rushing across pale skin.

I begin where I end.

I long to finger the outline of my shadow, to will it onto
   these walls,
to know it with clarity like a fact.

But we do not have the capacity to come to know
   ourselves in this life until the world uproots us, forcing us
   to commence again, with only the immaculate vision of
   hindsight to guide us, rolling us backward and forward in
   time, the documents of our being unbound, unbindable.

Womb—
I study this body of mine pocked with bruises and scars,
   this horror of mellifluous beauty,

this austere text of trauma and survival scribbled across my
   right side.

Do you know how precious you are?

Womb—
I close my fingers over my chimera, my echoing elusive
   memory of my past.

I find it.

I lose it.

Womb—
we are here, then too hastily ripped from the womb of life.

Oh, the humming whiplash of being alive right now.

I strain to stare at the cryptic choreography of sun on
   grass,
the swift squeak of birdsong painting air, a fading portrait
   vital and raw caressing sky,
perfuming atmosphere with jerky silence, wordless poetry.

Womb—
I wish to redraft the air, the broken vessel of my body.

But as long as I am still here,
I am still sacred,
still unsettled, still roiling and
rippling with the paradox of being human.

Oh, my right side, how my darling heart
kindles for you a lullaby, a candle flickering with
   recollection.

We all must surrender to endings out of sight,
unforeseeable, unshakable.

For even the tree lets go of its leaves yet endures, erect or
    bent, its gaze
fixated skyward, eternally looking at the heavens for
    direction.

Womb—
I contemplate my former self, a remembered chorus that
    aches with what was.

My stroke cannot steal this hushed whisper of self-
    cemented within.

Womb—
I must train this gentle voice into one of present
    emergence.

Womb—
this page is holding my hand, profoundly reaching into me
    for these words,
light bent into language grazing the darkness of my
    anguish.

Come be my companion as we break this exile, my lone
    voice harmonizing with yours,
as we eye in awe the light fall and catch itself in the womb
    of Earth.

Womb—
the glitch in my stroke, the token of a door with hinges
    wide-open.

We are all flourishing compost for worlds unimaginable.

I want to fly through air strumming my music across its
   atomic parts.

Womb—
I am a mortal broken creature.

I can no longer afford to resent and resist my afterlife.
I am a reluctant recipient of this situation, this unending
   ending.

But my stroke is my womb, my tuning fork to find myself.

For we were here the entire time unnoticed,
   unacknowledged, clawing for attention
we are not attuned to hear until the universe alters its
   slant,
manipulates the volume of silence.

Silence will find us all as we each come undone in own
   particular ways.

Even silence is mortal, vulnerable to wounds in itself, not
   with noise but with another
flavor of quiet-
an exhale, a sigh, a hug from within of my entire faulty
   nervous system,
a beloved fallen soldier fighting for air, for future moments.

I am a nocturnal tableau, an adapting, writhing, irate, real
   and undeniable organism of now.

I do not know what to do with the profusion of episodes
   of myself-

I am my own dead-end.

I no longer concuss against the truth of this body.

Womb—
abrasive distance of sudden trauma straightens the
    crumpled cloth of the world into refined,
clear truth, devastating and stunning light streaming
    through stained glass.

Womb—
sky my only ceiling,
grass my only ground.

Womb—
I lift my face to the tremulous voice in my soul I no longer
    fear, eager to extract and bottle it,
a mighty fire in the darkness, perhaps hope's new
    brushstroke.

I am alive, no matter how splintered.

I will make a womb out of the shape of these shapeless
    days.

Womb—
through the funnel of despair, I will birth myself
    undaunted, as I shed who I was and
define myself, greeting the world with a subtle smile.

Because life is not, nor was it ever, against me.

Life supports me, you, our union, our communion with
    these words.

Vulnerability

I once skimmed across the boundary layer of existence,
  cruising from one goal post to the next,
spellbinding myself into the lovely falsehood that I was like
pages of a classic novel forever bound
by leather ready to withstand vicissitudes of time,
that I was exempt from major
plot twists I did not choreograph.

Chronic illness stirred
me into my own mortality,
landing me bedridden at age ten
for months with the
biting sting that I could not outsmart life.

But, in that frame of being,
I was granted respite—
interludes of offloading innocence,
breaks in the stream of sickness,
instances that empowered me
about my body's resilience.

The fire in me remained bold and brash,
as tensile as it was in my
prelude cherubic years
during which death was merely a word,
not an eventuality,
an inevitability on reserve
for the elderly,
who are somehow born dying.

Now, as this pouncing predatory
spinal cord stroke
craters into my soul, life has turned its spine on me.

Resilience stripped itself of its bounce,
its definitional comeback,
is now pared back
into indiscernible white noise.

I presumed hardship emblazoned
itself on my being when my
cervical spine decided to destabilize,
when my arms and legs erupted out of joint.

But I knew nothing of this
pitched human
rocky terrain back then—
oh, picturesque menacing hindsight.

Perhaps I knew a smidgen.
Perhaps I had a taste.
But now, it occupies my entire pallet.

I am 28 but am really only one—
one year out since my life was derailed,
since I learned that I must learn how to
scamper along the tightrope
between life and death,
hanging onto the bleeding edge
of sharp vulnerability.

Show me another person who does
not know when she is thirsty,
hungry,

in need of a restroom,
how to walk,
how to breathe without her oxygen nosediving,
how to sit up without assistance,
how to dress and bathe herself,
and so many more mundane essentials
that add up to function,
that sweet causeway to independence.

There is no textbook,
no CliffsNotes I can analyze
to come up to speed on myself,
to comprehend my circumstances
and how they compromise me,
how they circumscribe me,
how they compress me into the
crib of forgotten self.

No number of scientific articles
will elucidate insight
into the depths of my mind as it
touches bottom and crouches there,
browbeaten in the dark.

The phone wires of my central nervous system
have been cut,
the cord severed between right and left—
the passage for direct connection
breached.

I am cloistered within myself.

My attempt at solace is a glass of soda that sits, initially
    effervescent

as I take refuge in my breath but soon fizzles out,
nightmares of unreal unreality revile me at my meditation's
    end.

If there were meaning here to find,
I promise you, I would locate it.

If my mother taught me anything,
she educated me how to vitalize
existence with significance.

But my suffering is no mask.

My hardship and loss are not cupboards I can open to
locate missing ingredients I seek.

Sometimes, the sadness prevails.

Sometimes, the quest for meaning
slips out of feasibility,
is blotted out by the gag of disability.

Oftentimes, fear triumphs—
the smoldering ashes of my once fantastical existence
get caught in my throat as normal conversations
between friends on street corners
elicit hailstorms of grief and despair.

When will words be sufficient again to tell my story, to
    make amends of nonsense?

Will they ever again hold as much muster as they once
    did?

I need to believe in words,
to be repatriated into syllables, more than anything else.

For if I can devote myself to words, I could perhaps begin
  to
reinstate faith in myself.

Floating

Here, immersed in these destination-less waters heavy with salt and darkness, I am carried where I need to go: out of time, out of space, out of illness, lifted off the rug of reality, risked head-first into a wormhole where everything, save for the roaring yet compassionate balm of silence, surrenders to stagnation, to the resounding thrum of the universe catching its breath.

Who is to say what the purpose is of it all?

Who can tell me that this very moment swaddling me in what feels like a serene millennium of tears is not what I was made for?

Who can say I mourn for myself in solitude when the water is crying with me, beside me, and beneath me, petitioning me for nothing but to permit me to feel my way through my feelings, to let them amass at the base of my throat and spill fourth, not with the goal of understanding but with the intent of being with myself as I am.

I tell the fear it can come forth out of its hiding place.

I tell the sadness it no longer requires the varnish of joy.

I tell the pain that I am ready to feel it all, to disassociate from disassociating.

I tell myself that being disabled does not equate to being unworthy of this life.

I tell myself that right here beside me you and everyone who has
ever

lived is holding my hand and mourning too.

Sonata

You and I plaster over fear,
drowning it in the sea of cascading thoughts,
in renewed charged cycles of our own undoing.

We fail to inquire within,
subconsciously
stoking the fire
catching in our brains.

What should have been momentary
trepidation gathers momentum,
expands until it chokes us,
enslaves us into thinking
it is the shape of our identities.

But my spinal cord stroke
stirred a swerve of consciousness,
guiding me into the knowledge
that fear is but the memory of pain.

I am grounded in this dilapidated body
depleted of sensation on the right side,
pulsing with agony and numbness.

In this very breath,
I am drinking a blend
of life and death.

So are you.

For this exact precious breath,
you will never breathe again.

This fragile moment is
waiting for you,
a dining reservation for which
you are remarkably late.

I only just showed up,
permitting the archives of mind
to turn up the quiet,
to turn down the volume,
the cadence,
of regurgitated thoughts,
doors opening into
to puddles of
disorienting grief.

Let us open a window.

Here I am.

I am ready for whatever comes next—
overloaded platefuls of despair
I will grapple with,
but never completely,
assimilate,
unanticipated emergence
from tragic suffering,
for the tangled,
twisted web of life
to catch me,

or push me down,
at its whim.

In becoming attentively still,
constrained by disability,
I am retrofitting
a new pattern of
internal freedom—
how to grow myself
within the unblinking eyes of trauma
into someone no longer afraid of fear.

Bless us as we prioritize words
that frame our faulty beings—
out of balance,
out of beliefs,
out of mainstream,
out of thriving,
as we are repressed and suppressed
with the gravity of questions
that tension us into unbound beings
too keenly present in the lax
socket of mortality,
inside the insight that we have
no wings,
nor did we ever,
but that we can rewrite
some of our sorrow
into the sonata of song,
that we can fly if only we
divert our constrained definitions,
so that words can converse

with our fractures.

We can hope.

We can even ride the
locomotive of childhood
inside the shock
of our disabled
bodies.

We are whole.
We are tarnished.

This is the rooting
from which we begin.
Vacillations

Time retreats—
I am a fly locked in its ember,
imprisoned in undying presents,
dreaming about running away from fraught strings of
    tenses,
tuning forks that turn me into dissonance with myself.

Tomorrow is a stream of syllables brutally neutered of
    meaning-
its once beauteous contours evaporate into garbled din,
unleashing a corrupting eruption of fireworks inside relics
    of my past,
expanding until it occupies the full cavern of my neurons,
brimming me with tears behind the barbed-wire fence of
    what was,
a word that brought beneath the telescope of
    consciousness

scorches the inside of my skin,
branding me with the sharp emptiness of the future
once as a part of me as my left arm now is.

Our lives are not the sagas we want them to be,
not the paragraphs we presume
we parse into publication within our being.

For this life is too feral and wild to be curtained off by
any sort of exoskeleton—
by words that are
too small and vapid
to structure the
profound profusion
that pours forth from the
harsh and miraculous everything that is.

Inhale and half your life is gone.

Exhale and you hazard flying away.

Nothing in this life is stripped of risk,
no matter the strategy deployed.

We are pilgrims at crossroads between being and
    becoming-
between enmeshing and emergence.

My parts fall out of me-
out of the right side of my being
I no longer feel since my stroke joined forces with my
connective tissue disease to correlate
sunrise with dislocations.

The beautiful breaking of morning holds hands with my
   mournful breaking.

This is the unshakable heart-wrenching elegance of being
   human.

I am, we are, balanced
on the fringes
of finitude,
a pile of fallen leaves-
on the cusp of turning yet unseen hues,
on the brink of erosion.

We never know when our own light will flicker out into
   darkness that predated us,
that will be our epilogue.

My despair succumbs to fuming rage as I claw through
   brambles and marshes of undoing suffocating sorrow
   and lament. I have been cruelly curtailed,
a canvas Monet only partially completed—
where is the start of the doctorate in genetics,
the first boyfriend,
the first breakup,
the lineup of unpredictable
jolting joys and anguishing agonies of this life?

Give me back the edges of my right side.

Give me back the contours of words.

I never know for whom my imperatives are intended, if
   they are only words hanging together in an internal fog

I am feeling my way through with the feeling still intact
on my left side.

I vacillate between a desire to yield to the armament of
trauma loaded with limitless ammunition and to adopt
Yates' yearning to bless to be blessed.

And, for some unreasonable reason,
I often wonder how that tree survives winter without
novels
to press into alternative lives-
meager but mighty literary mercies
that offer escape valves out of the
lengthy labyrinthine limbs of loss—
and this strange thought wraps me in the
warm embrace of gratitude.

I hunger to paint over interior walls of memories blanketed
with the
weight of unshakable truths.
This spinal cord stroke is a merciless educator who
constantly upbraids and thrashes its whip across my bare
flesh crusting with blood.

I thirst to live and live until I am no longer alive,
not to be the one whose heart resumes its steady rhythm
in the aftermath of a trauma that nearly bankrupted me of
breath.

I yearn to be lit up,
ignited by the ugly and beautiful transience of being-
for winter to spill into icy gusts into my chest,
to whisper into the ears of the word and crack open the
stale silence,

to leave a mark on this existence rather than being
   punctuated by it
with purposeless painful periods that end me before I
   even began,
to let me smell the fresh dew-
the newness of the world draining time wash over my
   body—
to be that whirlwind of curls again,
to be kissed a million times by rain,
to be burnt by blazing summer suns,
to feel the world's cursor glide across my skin.

And, most of all, I need to be joined in this forbidden
   furlough from freedom,
or, even more so, to be unchained from its manacles so I
   can join you-
so we can blur together into belonging and climb out of
   the confining carapace
in the invisible corners of the universe only felt and seen
   by the disregarded disabled.

Blessed

There is the taste of beatific forgetting,
enduring but for a truncated moment—
a magical splinter between webs of dreams and waking,
amnesia of the soul during which unreality glides through
   my fingers.

Suddenly, I am remade into wholeness, unbroken and
   unbreakable,
swiped clean of the crucifying stroke.

In that brevity of time between tangled darkness and
  benevolent light,
I am restored into the innocence of eternal youth,
into reflexive strength of my sense of safe certainty,
into someone who ate textbooks as though
understanding itself were a needle threading through
  nature.

This fraction of a second clothed in fog is a beautiful fuel-
an essential cog in the wheel that propels me onwards.

But, as sun seeps into slumber,
I arise undone—
with right ribs, a hip, or a shoulder lurching out of joint.

I am learning to let go of the steadiness I once implicitly
  presumed held the world together. For this universe
  is built of brutal uncertainty, commandeering us to
  capitulate as we encounter rancid fear while peering
through whorls tears into the unknown—
the million speakable and unspeakable
terrors that furrow into us until they feel as
stitched into our composition as our bones.

I yearn to staunch the flow of grief by curating and
  breeding my own brand of optimism, a blend I will test
  until it becomes a feeling I can grow into, a ladder I can
  emerge up and out from the shackles of jaw-clenching
  pain, despair and steep darkness. The loss accompanying
  disability is a hurricane, an everlasting unmaking of
  self that quakes through palatial tiles I meticulously
  constructed out of merit and grit, a delusion of luck
  veiled.

But that soon-to-be future I fallaciously
deemed a fait accompli recklessly riled against my
    naïveté—
inverting my body and my world
until it metastasized beyond recognition,
excluding me from experience,
landing me flat on my back,
stretched beyond the limits of bearable hardship.

I am the doll houses of my childhood tossed upside
    down—
dismantled worlds defying and defeating gravity to
    Newton's dismay.

I hunger to be blessed, despite my disinclination towards
    the God I inherited,
to feel my father's palms holding my head steady-
as though he could contain the calamitous catastrophe
    confiscating me from myself- as he whispers a
    benediction into my ear that everything will be alright,
even though we know it never will again be,
because the hugging softness of his voice is
precisely what I need to mitigate the pain,
the fear,
the absurdity of my own unraveling,
to glimpse something like a rainbow,
a miracle for an ephemeral slice of apocalyptic time
    in which I know with every blade of certainty I ever
    called mine that there are no conditions or stipulations
    associated with his undying love, that in all of my
    outlandish disability, I am enough with his firm yet
    tender grip holding my world still,

giving me everything I require to go on,
to hold on as I let go.

Conclusion

The speaker has catalyzed her passion for math and science into a poetics of self-reclamation as she rewrites the calculus of her past and present and discovers ways to incorporate a new math and science into her poetry.

Movement V
Lux

Introduction

The speaker's dialogues with the era before her stroke—the intimate stranger of her body, herself, and with her reader—grow more powerful throughout this section. Her poems alchemize into a call to change, to allow herself to be changed by her experience and survival.

Photons

Atoms of light, discrete bundles of electromagnetic
    energy, luminosity adorning Earth,
tactile sign language as these delicate scintillating fingers
    comb their way through hairs of darkness, creating
    shadows that distance and displace us from the
comfort of self.

We are all radioactive isotopes on the cusp of giving
    fractions of self away,
electrons drizzling out of us.

We are all running on the fuel source of loaned time,
    temporary slivers of flesh.

We only perceive nature through the lens of light rays it
   rejects,
mistaking that leaf as absorbing green when it truly invited
   every other
partition of light's spectrum but green into its essence,
the inside-out narrative we tell ourselves.

Oh, the legerdemain of our eyes that misconstrue
   stagnation out of entropy,
out of photons' perpetual motion.

Photons—
this world waits for no one, not even for photons.

Photons—
quanta bidding me to abide, to scavenge unwatched,
   primal light from my incarceration within the firm bars of
   disabled flesh, as robust a barricade
against being as the skin of that oak.

I am still picking myself up from the hurling, blurring,
   whoosh of
a single moment of traumatic trance and transplantation.

Photons—
the turf caved wide-open underfoot. I ricocheted beneath
   the canvas of myself,
leaking photons through my descent into darkness.

Tell me not to grip envy when my future is now a bygone
   era.

I have been laid off by my stroke,
sharp scissors radically lacerating me out of my
   emergence.

Photons—
come locate me in this night, repopulate my shadows
    through this static black.

I want the universe to pull me in close again, to press me
    into myself,
a vintage talisman in its pocket.

Do not reside so many light years away from my being.
Draw near as furtive slits of my eyes gradually shut against
    the palm of the world,
this unfathomable massacre.
My library of quantum physics textbooks too rapidly
    exchanged for this infinite stack of tragedy and despair.

My skin shudders a smattering of goosebumps at my
    eclipse.

Photons—
the uninvited guest of memory, a slow trickle bursting into
    a steady downpour.
I am drenched on rain-slicked streets of my soul, petals
    plastered on pavement.

All falls apart in this sodden inner city.

Oh, the photons, the flicker of memory-
my mother's unfaltering watch over my faltering body in
    the
intensive care unit as my heart rate and oxygen saturation
    nosedived,
my father's choppy sleep against solid wood,
my body toggling between being and oblivion,
every cell waging a war to be.

Photons—
oh, the pain of exposure, a frisson of goosebumps erupts,
landmines on skin, as I recall the slopes, the peaks and
    valleys, of my body
before- incandescently independent of the banisters of my
    father's forearms.

My body, a split-screen, now harnessed to cells within my
right side that has forgotten how to feel, are reluctant to
    divide,
to regenerate wiring to my brain.

Let me illuminate the photons of my right side, so I can be
    untarnished, worm my
my way back into mutualism, following the footfalls of tree
    and lichen, with the world, with myself.

Photons—
I will bow at the alter of the universe, this disabled afterlife.

I want to inhale the entire pungent ocean.

I want the shape of my name to feel like my mother's hug
    again.

Photons—
please shed light on this sorrow.

Give me back a dollop of innocence—
fingers glued with jam,
a smile winking eyes shut with glee.

Photons—
expose more radiance than this evanescent flat gray light.

My body bumped, careened against a speedbump
   without a warning sign.
Photons dissolved, time sped up, crashed its wheels
that continue to spin upended
almost two years later.

I am left behind, defying doctors,
as I discover the outrageous entrepreneurship of survival,
on some remote threshold between no longer and not
   yet.

Photons—
I need you to fill me up.

My virgin, unadulterated body is water that is too filtered,
   depleting it even of itself.

I have become nondescript to myself.

Whose face looks back in the looking glass?

Who possesses that penetrating glance, that vacant
   expression?

Is it yours?

Is it mine?

Is it something shared?

The hyperbaric chamber, my over ground tunnel fixated in
   space, transporting me nowhere, raising my devastating
   oxygen levels as I breathe myself into
becoming- a flimsy winnow of a creature,
a speck of flesh churning in a sea of glistening sparkling
   stars,

photons light years away, but close enough to confer
  sight.

Photons—
pay attention, burrow your gaze into each bumblebee,
every mountain, this blade of grass.

It is all so transitory.

Do not miss it.

Be with me in this dawn.

Photons—
how multicolored these black letters can be, even behind
  the rickety gates, the creaky grates of disability.

Metaphor, my current version of dress-up on the body of
  vowels and consonants.

Photons—
tell me, what story begins at the beginning?
Do we not always retrace the path, backflip with verbiage?

Writing begins at the bleeding edge that compels the pen.

Photons—
this stroke, my precipice, my launchpad.

A poem does not demand a swarm of language but an
  infestation of
feeling, a vast symphony of emotions, a letting go of the
  leashes in the mind.

Photons—
pause to ponder, stay still with me, as we listen to specters
  of wan light twisting through this page.

We can hear their crescendo.

Hunker down in this silence with me.

Do not fear it.

Photons—
my only task is to have a slender serving of courage,
to learn from the first brave letter that volunteers,
drawing a verse, calling me into being.

Lantern

There is a fire immolating my spirit,
a torch kindling the ashes of my soul,
scuttling them into oblivion,
into wherever things go when they leave us
in darkness alone.
I have left myself in the lurch,
in the immeasurable spaces between stanzas.
I am extinguished yet have yet to go extinct.
There is a wan lantern still intact in this besieged body
shedding tears of light through a funnel of gloaming.
I am not sure what to expect—
of myself, of temporal order,
an unrequited visitor who seems to have left my room,
to be elsewhere,
to be anywhere, but here.
Yet I am still resisting the gnawing temptation
to succumb to my irresponsive right side.

The neuronal tips that once effortlessly

enervated the right of me in their magical staccato have
   iced over,
set into an insuperable frostbite.
I am dejected yet unexpectedly and irrationally tranquil,
no longer victim to the red-hot sun of biting anger,
because jaw-clenching ire is far too unforgivingly
   formidable.
I lean into the darkness,
into loving this undone body,
no matter how much of me I can no longer
commandeer or transcend.
Perhaps life was never mine to transform at all,
not even in the before untarnished valley of becoming.
Perhaps that was the massive delusion,
this upside-down the authentic unadorned cavity of
   mortality
where I might seek home,
where I might locate the crucible within.
I am marshaling every molecule of courage
for anything to take root that
resembles being in my before,
because I am homesick
for that known lost clip of existence.
Call it foolish.
Call it delusional.
Call it whatever you wish.
All I can tell you is that something on the
inner creases of my skin is smiling,
pressing back at entropy,
unwilling to give me up,
unwilling to give in.

I will try on as many
healing stories for size as I can,
pairs of shoes at a store,
until I locate one that magnetizes
towards my inner compass,
my meek yet resilient lantern,
waiting with patience for verbal reservoirs
that fill me and that I can grow to fill.

Rewriting calculus

Hope is a cosine wave, peaking at the origin- the nexus
  between being and not being,
the launch-point of life, or, perhaps, beforehand in your
  mother's womb,
your father serenading you with homespun melodies,
your mother humming tales from books you have yet to
  behold, you have yet to fathom.
Too often now, I am mired in moments vanquished of
  language- inebriated by explanations that fall short of
  explaining the quagmire that is me.
My body- a rundown engine incompatible with self-
  sufficiency, excluded from throngs,
convicted of misplacing hope.
But that is, actually, the inversion of, or, maybe, but a
  fracture of the truth-
hope has stolen itself away from me.
I recurrently revisit my curated past—
I am seduced, disqualified,
brooding, reviled, reluctant,
ready to remake myself right here.

Hope is born before you are, before reality checks in. Hope's effortless and exuberant lance punches star-shaped holes in the dark bowl of the night—before the Big Bang, before atoms, before dinosaurs, before pain, before conjecture, before ignorance, before silence.

Hope churned the galaxy. There was a crescendo before you even knew who you were, what the world was, that you were in the world and the world was in you. Like the cosine wave, hope is a tide, the basketball I dribbled over stretches of New York for no reason other than to feel the discourse of rubber with fingertips, gravity working superlatively. But with each peak, rest assured, reader, I apologize to caution you: there is a nadir, sometimes as bottomless as self-exile. With each surge, there is a devastation, a demolition, a blackout. Hope is tempered, lost, neglected, abducted from you like the children you will never have because a geneticist notified you at 18 that having children is outside the confines of your anatomical possibilities, because at 28 you were struck down by a lightning bolt of a stroke, and with that stroke the last 28 years of your life were ripped away, wrapping paper haphazardly disposed of, and with that balled-up debris, hope was escorted out of you as though it had never been there, as though it had never known your name, as though you never smiled, never laughed, never dreamt, never held hope by the hand.

Reader, I am splitting hairs as I aim to co-opt my current feelings—

to override my despair, to convince myself that I once was something other than this runaway night. This thing I do—hurling words against the white page is idiotically the most terrifying but the most purposeful task in which I engage: stirring, finding rhythm, falling into puddles of words that drown me, slaughter me, never exposing just the right angle of my silhouette, and then, just as maddeningly, I ascend a scaffold of letters—my being tenderly held by its limbs,

by this heap of language—at once at a remove and so picturesque a spotlight—

at one in the laminate seam of poetry that domesticates trapped feelings.

If you search for affectation or terse encounters, you have unfortunately come to the wrong venue. I am elementally myself—

radially resected to the raw bones of who I always was, am becoming, smothered in humanity

as I toggle between keen insight and total engulfment

in the convulsions of trauma's headlock.

That is the conundrum of shimmying into greater proximity to language—

you shuffle out of it, loose your grip,

your lantern flying out of focus—you fail to see the light you cut.

But here I am over and again straddling ill-fitting words, entirely at a standstill how to aptly complete most sentences, how to make them sweep once more, lace in wind.

Let me know if you discern something in this hydra,

a weed developing I am too close to admire.

Hope was something you, former Elly, carried with you all the time. Hope was something you did not have turn in, be graded on, forget or figure out. It cosseted you. It defended you and girded you. It embraced you, and you did not even know it was there, aside from that smile,

those dimples flashing across your face that told you that hope

could go by so many names,

perhaps even an infinite number

or at least a multitude.

Hope lost its resurgence, a balloon deflated, hollowed of air, the ball no longer launching upwards and kissing fingertips. Where have you gone, dear invisible, and overlooked soulmate? What road have you taken that I have not? Did my stroke sink you just as it deafened my right side, ripping me into my disabled body, landing me in shambles?

Come back, be my cosine wave again. I do not need you to drive me over the moon as you once did—to prompt me to dance for no reason,

to pump fists in air at the sheer bliss of being.

I do not expect that much of you, or anything, at this bitter juncture. But I need you in my life. Disability does that; it definitionally renders you distressingly dependent. Bring me a few rays of weak light. Bring me some levity in this nocturnal slant of being.

Reader, be with me in this surreal downpour of despair—

hope tipped inside out.

I need to hold you, reader, on the other side of these words, so that we encircle them,

let them settle in my marrow for a while, for their truth weighs on me alone too mightily. I need you to be with me at its panting pulse. But there is no need to over-grip here. Success and failure are not working binaries boxing us in any longer. That is a trembling blessing of disability—the discipline of being morphs into a fog you need not transcend. Let us be humble and subtle here in our betrothal to support. Let us repose to observe, or, better yet, to rewrite, another waveform, pen courage into and around it, so our frontline fears flatline as we thaw a yet unknown fulfillment of hope.

Cross-Pollination

There exists perfuse feeling in numbness,
dappled light shimmering beneath veiled eyelids,
dynamism in immobilization,
microscopic pores in clenched fists,
compassionate tickles under choked tears,
shafts of hope in rooms crowded with despair,
communion with air in solitude,
intermittent fringes of smiles in desiccated sadness worn
    and primordial,
presence in the absence of everything you once thought
    true.

For everything on this planet mingles with everything else, even when the two contradict each other blatantly.

We cross-pollinate.

Will you dazzle me with a bit of your pollen—
a syllable or comma-
so I may whorl out of myself?

I will find myself in self-evacuation.

I will hide, and I will seek.

Will you join me?

The game of life—
volleys of chance that mangle you until you slip off cosmic
    wallpaper—
are perhaps vacuums for you to fertilize so you emerge
    again,
rather than bluster into an object of pity discarded by
    tragedy.

We cannot alter the raw bones of truth, but we can array
    them—
pile adverbs and adjectives to highlight and dog-ear who
    we are, how we are—
subtle dials of parallax that shift everything and nothing.

Let's change the word, and not a single subatomic particle,
    together.

Restrain any urge to chaperone me into generalizations-
flimsy and narrow stereotypes that expand the perhaps
already expansive space between us,
to elevate, supersaturate, your self-worth above
subversive categories you bracket me inside.

Instead, let all of your declarative assumptions
dilate into questions unbound by constructs.

Engage with these words so they undefine me,
pummel you out of limitations you impose.

I am learning to exude this breath I have been holding for
    over
a year since a doctor made a grave mistake,
inking a cervical cord and medullary injury
on this body that we all end with, end in.

Why must every pound of meaning dissolve with our
    pounds of frail flesh?

I want to be the person who refuses to relent to the
    crushing brutality of it all.

I do not seek to retrace my steps, to reclaim a past into
    which I no longer fit.

All I aspire to do is to keep breathing,
keep writing and rewriting everything I tell you and myself.

Do not expel my words, but swallow mouthfuls of
my clang and clamor, my anguish and devotion.

Even with this poem, no matter the Olympic gymnastics of
    metaphor,
I will never successfully transfer me into you,
into the shape of thoughts,
but it is your choice to let my words not only
pass through but transform you.

My body, my mind, my story are, alas, my own.

So are yours.

That is the magic, the misfortune of mankind.

If only I could share it all for a spell.

If you yield to temptation to place me in a box, rest
   assured,
I will find a way, a street grid, out.

Because if I am still here-
these words rebounding off dimensions of my sick room,
I am not yielding to any binaries or to
the victim-status malpractice chiseled at the upper-
   echelon of my spine.

We harbor more agency than we accredit ourselves.

We cross-pollinate kinship of recognition.

You can briefly see me at eye-level through windows of
   tumbling words
before returning to your level-ground.

If I am uttering these words,
molding something out of nothing, I can simmer in how
   things are.

Will you taste and eat these words with me as we perform
   the most human duty-
drafting and redrafting our stories?

Everything is happening.

All I have to do is be.

Be with me.

I am scouring my dark hardship for all of the light I cannot
   yet see.

Spine

The instrument that ties us into being,
wires us into a network of towering vertebrae,
the anchoring trunk that branches us into projections of
   limbs,
a creaky stairway,
a vertiginous highway,
a frail yet stoic byproduct of millennia of inheritance and
   genetics gathering steam in me, in you, as we veer
   sharply,
align our bodies on shadows of trees.

My algorithm of self now growls,
now a source of immense pain,
once an invitation to be in direct communication with
   nature,
with the status quo,
now a taunt as doubt backflips through lacunae in my
   spine,
landing me unmoored from the dock of what was as I
   clatter through
existence in another's skin.

Why does inevitability always intrude too soon?

How hasty the drop from ordinary to catastrophe.

Spine—
I beseech you to yoke me back into myself,
to simultaneously root me and permit me to reach
   heavenward.

Oh, what a blessing unrealized that was-
to possess an intact spine, a united bulwark against the
    menacing world.

Let give myself once more
to speed,
to the crisp breeze,
to tumbling through mud.

Spine—
give me back this sacred pillar of body,
this wondrous axis of symmetry past,
not long ago as tense and unbroken as a violin string.

Spine—
my body lapsed out of order,
a spinal cord injury shredding feeling out half of me.

I am now the sentry of my right side deleted from my
    brain,
as though it were but a redundant
line of this verse
extinguished,
unnecessary.

But I am a bipedal human,
an outgrowth of Darwinian evolution,
I long to cry into the rift in my universe.

I hunger to lilt in fields of sun-soaked tulips,
to gallop aimlessly through brambles, pavement, grassy
    hills
until a smile stretches itself so wide across my
    countenance it hurts,

mopping my cheeks with falling tears at the light beauty
  of being.

I long to prance after moonlight dancing on water,
to fall into step with others, with myself,
on a right foot I can
once again
feel.

Spine—
oh, how absence of sensation on my right half roils
  through me.

Oh, how darkness leaps, telling me my somber saga over
  and again, inflicting traumatic pain over and again, the
  never-ending past igniting my present with malevolent
  electricity.

I watch my old self falter as these syllables arch towards
  what was,
raw vowels alchemizing into swooning wisps of memory
  and desire.

Spine—
we are all held in captivity of mind.

We can stand together
separate from logic and
common sense.

Your disabled body, your upbraided soul, can accompany
  me and mine.

Please do.

My past is deep underwater,
left on its own, elsewhere.

Is yours?

Spine—
night hugs me tight, its searing grip all too firm—
I hear my tender bones crackle, my chest a balloon
    deflated of air.

The dark is choking me.

How dense is your night?

I am a tourist, not even a tour guide, in my inventory-
the museum of my before,
the Smithsonian of my soul.

Spine—
in stark desiccated silence, my cry is a lantern.

I am a million
empty
echoes.

Can you hear me?

Spine—
air roars, trembling and terrified.

I thirst to rock the spine of my youth in my arms.

Spine—
let me press reset, even if I need to hold the
button for eternity
plus an
hour.

How can you go on?

How can you give yourself away?

Spine—
my once halo, the gilded rim
of my nervous system, in which I am now an
outlaw, indicted.

Why?

I scream into the unanswerable hole in my broken body.

Spine—
I look within, a detective into my own history.

It is all too unsayable,
too ungraspable, too inescapably hard-
I have her earrings,
her clothing,
her toothbrush,
all of which I must screen my eyes against,
all of which feel like staring into the heart of a blazing sun,
possessions too immaculately preserved.

Spine—
dig me out of this melancholic stupor.

Give me back my
right boundary,
my right body,
my right factory settings.

Spine—
poetry is my mother, my uprooting from

time and space, my refuge into emotional imaginings-
chords of liquid gold spoken and seen,
my enduring spinal cord and sustaining sustenance that
    catches
at the cloth of your soul, snagging at its seams, fusing us
    into something
close to whole.

Close is enough for me.

Is close enough for you?

My name is being called by a force I cannot yet name.

Spine—
I am holding my broken body, embracing it with every
    molecule of love in this world.

Because it has taken me this long to take notice of the
    second word in broken open-
that my rending, my spinal cord stroke,
not only stole from my body but bequeathed me
an opening, a point of entry,
to hear the music of these words, my fishing line, my bait,
my becoming, my being.

Parachute

I persist on a borrowed visa, my right to be here called into
    question each day.
There is nothing about me in sync with the world,
with reality as I once knew it or as it knew me.
We were once on quite good terms.
But now, I wonder how I am that same person—

or even subsumed under the same species-
who used to wear this same skin and bones,
who used to harbor a panoply of gusto, charisma, and
    vitality, not this now splintered soul,
these too exposed nerve endings.
I feel as though I wear a costume each day or I am a
    Russian doll,
my nested incarnations of self-dislodging one at time.
Let me know if you see them on the road and have the
    strength to gather them for me.
I promise to pay you in words.
While I look the same without, someone else has taken
    residence within.
There is but a kernel of stamina left,
sufficient to confront my own barbed psyche on this page.
For what would I do if I gave up words, if the very particles
    of my mind exiled me like my former form? Would I
    disappear? How would I know I still existed?
How would you ever find me?
I have been swept out of my own narrative,
not even worthy of assuming the role of understudy, of my
    own one-woman show.
Tears skid down my cheeks as I overhear crumbs of
    normality, sudden breaks in the riptide of disaster- a
    mother exchanges blessedly with her son about his
    school day or schoolgirls meander down the sidewalk,
    skipping and laughing.
And here I am, this sideliner deprived of herself, this
    dependent disabled daughter ungrowing up. I have
    been ostracized in solitude in a desert.
The universe has become parched to me.

I fear the words as they hesitate to capture my suffering, to
    mop it up into legibility.
But I am more afraid of abandoning them, because
    otherwise, how will I know that I have not vanished, that
    I am still here? How would you locate me?
There is not much hope left in me now.
I have spent it all, an impulsive buyer at an outlet mall.
And I am lost, perhaps forever to the world, but not
    necessarily to myself.
For if I am writing, if I have the river of words and the
    infinite banks between what the words cannot say, if I
    have a morsel of faith in the black letters, I might have
    hope that the page will be my parachute, catching me
    over and again.

Lattice

In the basement of my soul is a lattice of tunnels
    culminating at a garden-verdant and wildly overgrown.

Trees respire alongside vines climbing heavenward.
Infinite networks of roots mingle, transgressing
    boundaries,
overlapping dynamic patterns of life over life, being
    overlaying becoming,
a constant flow of dynamism in darkness.

There is no light.
There is no water.
There is just this being fusing with becoming, unending
    fields of green mounted on stalks that give way to
    sunflowers and tulips as decorously blushing with

vibrant colors as any you may observe beneath a blazing sun.

But here, in this ramshackle habitat deep within my darkness,
the sun neither rises nor falls.

At least we are pardoned from observing the absent light depart.
Dear reader, grant me the gift of your palm without forcing me to say farewell.

Let's mine infinity here.

There is life.
There is an almost quixotic evolution in the presence of horrific trauma.

I permit the pain to grow me, to weave me into you.
I let the fear facilitate renewal without requesting the inevitably impossible of you,
the universe, or of whomever is in charge of anything,
to temper trepidation quivering in my bones.

I ache for grounding.

This stroke will be my sacrosanct garden,
seeds that will sow me into someone worthy of my trust.

I will not always surrender, to the best of my capacity,
to the temptation to claim the role of victim, which mine to claim at my own peril, at the risk of morphing into someone I despise, someone static in the muck of despair,
someone hopelessly on the verge of disappearance.

I need you to see me. Do not let me peter out of view.

In these words, I am encountering and watering myself, glistening green out of black ashes.

The light will never shine as it once did.
The leaves will never be tickled with water as they once were.

But, alas, the past is always past.

All I have now is a self to grow out of a nightmare.
Nonetheless, rebirth may transpire. Growth is happening in these words, in the chipped straitjacket of my stroke.

Something unbreakable is breaking through the dense thicket of trauma.

There is always a chance for something to take root.

Let's hazard ourselves.

I will till the soil of my soul until my arms relent,
even if it occupies the duration of my time here.

Rehearsal

Here is a beginning in darkness.
I perch on the edge of my seat in solitude as
close to my own consciousness as possible.
I muster the silent tenacity to tiptoe into each word,
gathering courage,
rare species of flowers on the ground,
to step into a right leg combed of feeling.

I dare not squint at the end of my story, nor even its
    middle,
but am content with beginning right here.

I gamble it all—every cent within my pocket of audacity—
not the antithesis of fear, but living adjacent to fear—
that smothering neighbor perpetually knocking on your
    door,
inking a portrait of knuckles on wood.

The stakes could not be higher.

I shirk any plea for fearlessness—
an unaffordable commodity
in this afterlife.

I leap into the eye of my own storm,
into my dismembered body in my brain,
into feeling too much inside my soul and
into feeling nil in my right corridors.

Each day, I surrender all
my savings—
renounce my past,
begin again with as much
adaptability as this besmirched
body can hold.

All I ever do is rehearse.

I am earning a PhD in practicing,
as I dabble in the abrasive
education of suffering.

All you ever do is rehearse,
even if you are not aware of it,
even if you resist the thought.

I practice ordering words so the maelstrom of disability
does not overcome me—
fails to leave me raked of my residues,
treading the broken thoughts of my own brokenness.

If I write,
leaning into the
pen tacked to my throat,
I am here,
resoundingly and resolutely present
as my words prickle your lips.

I write to exorcise the experience,
to whittle down this pain into a size
that can fit neatly within my body
without spilling everywhere.

I mop up this hurt with these metaphors.

Unfortunately, there is no right image
that can distill and concentrate this dagger
of a young stroke into a nectar of gilded metaphor.

There is but this swarm—
a meteor shower of metaphor—
for you to shuffle and
determine what grips you,
what reflects and refracts
from this out-of-focus whirling
collection of pocket-sized

images I hurl onto this white page,
onto you to see what sticks.

I practice walking on my derelict right leg,
hoping the kinked, crossed signals in my
central nervous system will one day synapse connectivity,
however tenuous,
between brain and body.

These black and white letters loosely
hung together into porous imperfect sense-
my graffiti on the wall,
my hydrographic on interior caves—
tell me I am here.

I wonder still about that girl who dazzled
before a brainstem injury and cervical cord trauma
   dawned on her,
locking her out of her once immaculate life, the key firmly
   securing the lock,
and dream smooth dreams of where she may be.

If I shut my eyes, I see her perusing clothes at a nearby
   shop.

Let us close our eyes and serenely bless her.

Let us bless everything we can bless.

I feel her finger scanning spines of books at her favorite
   bookstore.

She is almost excruciatingly real.

She is embedded in my mind.

I live in jaw-clenching pain.
I live with immense loss,
in the tense,
bony elbows of trauma.

I do not know if this saga has an ending,
or even a middle.

So, all I can do is begin every day,
is take the giant,
silent step of faith into this vulnerable moment,
into this premeditated breath,
into this staggering syllable slicing space.

Because when I encounter my own consciousness,
I migrate to outskirts of the tattered quagmire
of my body that no longer knows
sight in my right eye,
hearing in my right ear,
unthought ease of swallowing,
and a riptide of other biological features that
stood up and walked across
the barricade opened by my stroke from
subconscious to all too conscious.

The velocity of the hurt slows,
nearly fades into oblivion,
when before me I only see the necessity of rehearsing-
a white page and alphabetical tapestry that do not note
the shape of my body but only trace migrating contours of
  my soul.

Watercolor

Tell me, where does my right-side end and reality begin?

Where do you end or begin, if you end or begin at all?

What about the caterpillar on that tree bark, that pigeon
    soaring overhead?
Do they even flinch at the thought of their particular
    cutouts in the scheme of nature?

Why must we be so alone with ourselves in the
    electrifyingly unfeeling cosmos
when we are all one with the natural world- conversing
    with it in silently mellifluous exchanges of oxygen and
    carbon dioxide,
a barter system yielding mutual rebirth.

For even our deaths are living ones, sources of fuel for
    organisms underfoot.

For when we die, we are but returning home for the first
    time,
burrowing into blissful stability beneath the breathing
    Earth.

I have become the watercolors I used to paint,
the right half of my body I can no longer sense bleeds into
    everything,
seeping into man-made structures, into the natural
    habitat,
rendering me incomplete but not alone,
my impermanence manifest in every movement attempt
    on my right side,

to which I whisper in hushed tones, as though it were a
    child I newly adopted,
something unaccustomed to me, something that now
    blends into everything
because everything spills into everything ultimately, at
    least.

So I beseech myself to tear down all of the barriers I can,
to rise up from the familiarity
into unanswerability.

Because in this after,
I yearn for my soul to leak as well,
for the rhapsodic sublime to drench me in a downpour of
    my own becoming.

Perhaps then, I can migrate, a wren perched on a branch,
from being victimized to being with whatever is.

In solitude, I am susceptible to hear the rumblings of my
    soul as
its feet creek along the floorboards
of the one part of me that cannot be unmade by trauma.

I am not aspiring in the direction of answers.
For life has chastened me, has whipped me with its
    grueling belt buckle
on the raw skin on my back, that existence is insoluble.

But I have learned, through the petrifying puberty of pain
    and grief,
that my soul knows how to sing.

I am slowly teaching myself how to listen to every note,
etching a language out of the unsayable.

Evanescence

Vaporous wisps evaporating into forgetfulness, into
   loopholes in memory,
fine mist on a windowpane rapidly condensing back into
   its cloudy home on a summer day, the impermanence
   predominating each heartbeat, any inhale,
this run-on sentence of presence, every existential hum
   vibrating through the atmosphere, that stoic pine just
   beyond my field of view.

For even the darkness itself, every atom in this cosmic
   scheme, comes undone.

Evanescence—
I fall out of the illusion of control, a spell cast unraveling.

Evanescence—
horses cantering, dispatched across countrysides into
   pitch black night,
into dreamscapes, into relics of fevered thoughts you
   cannot remember,
reveries that cannot remember you.

Disability: an enforced abstinence from the world- is
   abusive master.

Gallop me back to the annals of past,
to limitless timelines,
itineraries you scripted as a six-year-old
swinging in Tennessee.

Evanescence—

my stroke dissolves me, one painful particle at a time, of
   myself.

I grimace at the autobiography of my right side I no longer
   perceive
through layers of tears.

Direct me how to direct a life with only half a body singing
   to my brain.

Evanescence—
watch me as I disappear, a full eclipse overtaking the sun.

Evanescence —
I catalog this overcast shadow of grief in the sinew of
   words.

But there is an abundance of raw feeling that cannot be
cut into words, that must be exuded and
expelled in the gaps and gasps between them.

Let us be with this interlude drenched in sorrow.

Let's let ourselves cry, ring ourselves out,
towels drying in blazing heat.

Evanescence—
permit this silence to linger, a vertigo of the soul as it
catches fire that relents and rises,
a dirge,
a song unsung,
a eulogy,
a lullaby,
a melody of rhapsodic poetry dipped in syllables poisoned
   in ivy of tremulous quiet.

Evanescence—
do not fear the echolalia of empty spaces, solitude
   predicated on this stroke of trauma.

Through the evanescent hours, I am holding your hand
   lovingly, as we-
intimate strangers accustomed to the thrift of existence
   born of brutal vulnerability-
hold fast to these evolving transparent words sparking
   with electricity.

Evanescence—
academics dropped away—
the fruits of my almost three decades of toil, of seeds
   planted,
judiciously plowed without the privilege, the rightful
   outgrowth, of collection, purged without consent, my
   future confiscated by the thorny tentacles of trauma
   ossifying into disability, a miasma of unreal proportions
   assaulting the entirety of my life.

Where did it all go—
that wondrous luminary logging her way through Harvard
   Yard,
her flowering social society-
her lost unlived days once so easily seen,
leaves swerved afield by unruly wind?

Evanescence—
a rending of body, an outcast in this echo-chamber of self,
   this master of nothing coming into someone she does
   not yet know is setting a new curriculum for herself as

I engage in dialogue with you across continents and
   oceans of suffering,
in conversation with previous versions of self in margins of
   books-
study steeped in the tender bones of humanity.

Evanescence—
let us be in this mortal penumbra unveiled to ourselves as
too fragile, too temporal, too ephemeral,
too evanescent without anodynes for being time-stamped
   creatures.

Let's find repose in each other, in these shattered bodies
   we do not want but, nonetheless, have.

With me, find gratitude in this hardship, in this knee-deep
   melancholy.

Evanescence—
let's find each other so that in harmony we mingle into a
   fractured whole,
our sharp edges visible but united,
beauty radiating from rupture, from the potency
   encapsulated within the excruciating
truth of what it means to be alive- evanescent organisms
   erupting into epic episodes,
into eventide, into eternity.
Liminality

The black bold line
between before and after—
a cumbersome harness into the
unforgiving grip of trauma—
who demarcated it,

etched it indelibly so
it slices
my skin and
draws blood?

I did not carve this chasm, sanction this undoing-
a barely bearable break in the flow of life.

Will I be found in this after?

Is there a frost coating my
eyes you recognize,
a mirroring glance that
speaks the crater of
lost language of loss,
whispering into the
concavity in your soul,
"I have been there,
to the upside-down,
inside-out,
tilted side of being.
I see you.
I hear the piles of unsayable words
and the pounds of vocabulary that
cannot hold your sorrow.
I feel you.
You are a treasured
shipwreck on the ocean floor,
but I am too"?

Grant us this ejected
fraught liminality—
the invisible in-between—

the shivering,
scalding fear of
embodying our own endings.

Will my before forever shoot through my mind,
a gun firing ceaselessly?

Will this dense
barrier thaw into
one dotted with
emptiness—
blank space
for me to fill
at my will—
acquiescing to
opportunity of becoming an ion
sliding across a membrane, ping-ponging between
what was and my nightmarish now?

I yearn for white space-
what cipher is written there?
What emotions have you stepped into there? -
for memories to crawl back-
that once uncropped smile,
that once unedited spinal cord.

My memory oscillates,
a mutating valence—overwrought by my current despair
   that
it is as though
my past has been
annulled, crossed out with red ink,
as if it were but a school paper

marked with totalizing failure.

Hum to me the salient fragments
of before, so I know I arrive
when,
if,
I am blessedly
authorized
to return.

Consolations

Right of the border of my spinal cord,
I fear the civilization of neural networks is corroding,
fading into oblivion,
a trailing off into
a once upon a time
Gilded Age.

I lull myself inside the thought that I still hear its steady
   whispering ionic exchange,
its consoling dynamic whistle across axons,
it's almost waltz that revved me up with
plentiful kinetic energy,
now muted and mutated into silence,
a petrifying purgatory pulsing with pause.

I want the alarm to go off at full blast,
to jive the hard drive enmeshed in neurons into action,
into excited saltatory conduction,
a tango with my central nervous system once more,
into a sense of my own sensation and proprioception

on a side of my body that has lapsed into a sabbatical of
    heavy silence,
a cup overflowing with emptiness.

Who ever thought that an absence could weigh so much,
that lack of feeling could be so intense?

I am in direct communion with the right side of my being,
locking eyes with it now so it remembers my name,
my biological geography,
my once giddy affinity for moving through the world,
    almost heedlessly,
my once unflinching trust in my own footing
that I need not look down to ensure my right foot kissed
    Earth.

I loved the implicit connection I shared with myself,
the recklessness I wore like a daily uniform as I meandered
    through nature
with a novel in hand, alternating between scanning tree
    branches and streams of sentences.

I miss that girl's unadulterated smile tugging at the corners
    of her mouth,
and I wonder where she has gone, if she has perhaps
    taken residence
within the right half of my being, which feels more like a
    hiding place,
more like a mannequin, than anything belonging to me.

She is in my, our, imagination mid-song,
in the first phases of gulping air into sonic creation,
her poetry lent the hand of melody,

trapped in weary recollection and creeping every so often
like a child's footfall on wood-
gentle, real, dissolving, just beyond the periphery,
always looming but too far out of view.

Help me lionize the Elly effect in you.

I fear the firefly of her blinking black against dark.

I want to draw you into the grace of her question I
now wear across my indefensible nervous system all the
    time-
her changing shadows on my walls,
her traces,
the clatter of her steps,
the production of her expressions—
how rapidly they washed across her now vacant face,
her gestures, piano fingers rippling through air
as she ranted about Richard Feynman,
how the mysterious universe made her feel
so preciously small,
exuberantly deliciously eager to color
each neutral moment in technicolor.

You see, I need to confide in you about
my vanished self, so you can spend a few days with her,
so I do not lose track of her in words as I did in life.

I do not want her to slip out of these slick blades of
    language.
I need her to squat here, so we can bide company with her
    for a while,
lease her mouthfuls of oxygen she never received.

She is my model. I fumble to reenact her here for you,
    desperate to canonize her so
you can access how spectacular she was,
she who once inhabited this now ball of knotted
    musculature.

What is this substantial silence she has left behind?

Can you hold its canopy with me?

My arms are growing numb and throb for you.

I yearn for these neurons to sing again,
to harmonize with melodies once descending
from my central nervous system.

Chant right side, ungrow back into your light dreamscape.

I feel so disconnected,
a phone off the hook, from myself.

Place me back in the receiver.

Let the sensation that evaporated long ago condense me
    back into unity.

Reader, be in this mesh of still quiet with me as we cradle
    the right side.

I mourn the now garbled language of my body.

I thirst to know its vernacular.

I will speak any tongue, even if it is that of silence,
if it means I can interact with this half of my being, this
    crater I refuse to abandon,

this womb of sadness and despair paramount to who I am,
who I can become.

Be in these fractured nuanced spaces with me,
as we bide time in taboo limbo.

I want to learn from this side of my being how to be gentle
and patient with myself,
how to be graceful in the face of a trauma I will never
overcome or metabolize fully,
how to be easy on myself despite the lapse in my ability to
override this hardship.

I am not software readily installed and uninstalled.

Are you?

My right side is teaching me more than I have learned
from anything else in this world.

I will become its apprentice for life, without expectation,
aside from the
possibility that it will permit me to cultivate myself
internally
into someone profusely perseverant with herself,
even if the sun never again rises as it once did.

Cauldron

There's a cathedral in my mind,
sanctuary in my soul—
an untapped cauldron,
bruised yet stoic,

disregarded in a secret cupboard locked from without for
   eras,
newfound artifacts I suspected snipped
along with the synapse wiring my brain to my right side.

I mourn the sensation strumming through my right interior I unwittingly possessed—that succulent soft mingling of skin against skin, that incipient experiment of contact: your mother's brush against your forearm. Yet this citadel of wholeness is underfoot—perhaps enmeshed in undergrowth. Perhaps I need to dig deeper, draw a bit closer to the source, mine it as if I were a quarry, enthralled to forge precious gems. I hazard the feeling that nothing remains, yet I opine that there's still something tucked beneath the surface—this stroke will always be mine until I am absent from this planet. I am distilling axioms—the raw why bones that I still am—because evolution aspires to exile us all from its genetics of chance, its gamble in favor of the fittest—a class with which I no longer feign affiliation because I veer so far astray from the bell curve of normal. I ache for my own distribution of extreme complication, extreme exasperation, extreme loss, and extreme disability—if only to localize myself within the soothing arms of statistics.

Yet, I am here—an organism limping into movement, into futility, and, intermittently, into a stalemate—a feat that ferments into a win when I can regain my visual bearings, tame the symptoms that haunt my mornings and evenings—the convulsions that shake my right arm out of its socket, lurching downwards, a fallen monolith that descends until my face encounters carpet. I refrain from screaming because I do not expect anything different at this point, after this seventh month hall of horrors.

I do not anticipate waking into sensing anything on my right. I even resigned from searching for it with my left arm or my eyes to ensure its ongoing existence. I am pared back to the simple-minded insight that all I can do is try—a locomotive ignited by extrinsic and intrinsic forces, a melding of my parents' devotion and inner grit that falters and recovers over and again, a case of bipolar seasonal allergies. I am not invested in rewinding time or in prescience. I am strengthening my muscle to be in now: between no longer and not yet, inside the discomfort of liminality, between feeling and not feeling, between relenting and persevering. I live in margins of journals pasted with words and books I burrowed into before my cervical instability advanced, was convoluted by my brain damage. There's yet room to persist, bountiful levers of hope to pull, something I do not have language to name to swaddle in belief, despite my nervous system's glacial healing. I am not the source—the tap bathing belief—but something steadfast, perhaps unvoiced and unvoiceable, tugs me forward though the lethargy of heavy hours despite the brute knowing that my universe folded in on itself like I were a poker game and you quit on me, you called my bluff. But I'm still playing, if not dealing the cards. I'm still reacting to life's redaction. My synapses leave ineffaceable ellipses of tears. For they too have lost their innocence, leeched of renegotiating connections to radio silent portions of me. Do not redact these unpolished words, my tears, or the counterpoints of white space sloshing between it all, between us—these nuanced pauses where we land, regather ourselves, return to the sacred flying buttresses of our internal cathedrals that no one, no matter their authority or maleficence, can decimate from who we can always become.

Diatomic

I wake into a pathless dark woods overgrown with thorny
   barbs,
into a disabled body attacked in elastic night—
a haze of lost ribs and limbs detour from anatomical
   capsules,
testing the agility of slack sockets that no longer seatbelt
the right side of my being into cohesive containment.

With Sisyphus' absurdity,
I inch fragments of self I no longer feel back into
   assemblage,
into the necessary illusion of oneness amidst
fierce formidable nullification.

Bind me up to my knees in sensation.

Steep me in less thought.

Show me my lineage—
the galloping beauty in this disproportionate being,
in this unstable misaligned organism doubled over in the
   screeching grind of pain.

Do not debase me for my wheelchair,
for the omissions running through your mind once you
   fixate your eyes,
only fathoming a fraction—
the false dichotomy whiting out your mind,
impulsively miswriting the dropped stitches of my story
   unreachable by eyes.

That is but your projection of you

onto my uncertain
package of skin and astray limbs.

If you are able-bodied,
this is your alarm clock—
you cannot unread me,
even you dare to scan this poem in reverse.

If you are in a parallel predicament,
I am sincerely sorry for your wounds,
but welcome you to find your
signature in mine.

I am a pastel drawing—
a dark contour once lucid that now
blooms into infinite shades of gray tending towards the
    white page,
deafened by fingertips smudging through lines,
effacing boundaries that render the sketch,
and my own wretched body,
obfuscated as to where its right side begins or ends.

You are suspended in the pinwheel of my words.

I am suspended in your silence.

We intervene,
interrupt,
complete each other—
two forces circularly landlocked in each other's inertia.

The logic of the world-
that only avidly existed within networks of mind—
has retreated like many of my past peers,

incompatible with this version of my being—
so excruciatingly vulnerable and mortal.

I reside in unending
wintertime grief leaching momentum
out of my bloodstream until my velocity dips
towards zero—
landing me in some shadowy purgatory,
an underworld cobwebbed with immobile trauma,
out of sync with my familiar—
the blessed hum of hurry,
the beautiful barrage of mundane tasks,
the bold articulations of two feet I could feel
venturing through marathons of movement.

Tell me, what does walking on two sensate soles feel like?

The memory is crawling its way out of me, welling me with
    tears.

The 15 months since my unmaking accost me like a
    fairytale era-
my decadently stratified Bach prelude redacted,
as though it were nothing more than drawing on
    whiteboard.

That girl came and left, disappearing without me.

I ache for a summation of all prior selves
to arrive within the elbows
of this moment-
for all of my previous appearances to knit together into a
    now.

But they do not.

I am partitioned from myself—
from key features of the person I deemed elemental to my
  emergence.

Can you dislodge romantic happiness too frequently,
rattling it into ambiguous limpness that it forgets its home
  joint,
its socket at the palpitating heart of you?

If so, can you regenerate that feeling, its landing strip, your
  total immersion in it?

Do not look through or around me.
See me for everything I am,
everything I can no longer be.

Let's imagine divergent lives together,
become bonded orbitals—
twin hydrogen atoms meeting,
embracing in diatomic deftness,
promising never to let go.

I wish I could filter this haphazard stroke out of me.

But this reality is not a granter of wishes—
does not come with an insurance policy in the event of
  existential exigency,
is not the guarantor we yearn for it to be,
is a matrix of ruptures of the selves we erect over and
  again,
sandcastles on the shorelines casting incredible shadows
as they are washed away without leaving a trace

of their once having been.

As I now have the time to scrutinize atoms of words,
it hits me that remembering is not synonymous with
    recalling—
does not entail a tethering of tenses, a hauling of past into
    presence,
but instead requires more bravery than any human
    undertaking.

It is precisely because I have been dismembered,
as my catastrophe quakes through my being,
shattering the floorboards of my interiority—
that I have come to realize that remembering
demands a self-gluing together into this yet unknown
    incarnation—
a door upon which I must muster the terrible tenacity to
    knock,
a painful piecing together of what permeates this after
    that has,
in all of its uproarious unmooring,
only brought me precipitously proximal to the brutal
    bones of
what it means to be human-
to being jettisoned out of yourself,
to reinventing yourself with the thorny wisdom that you
    will not last,
to waking to the vital futility of continually
re-membering yourself,
a process that will break you
and make you over and again.

And this stroke absented me of so many biological drives
I never before brought beneath the microscope of
   consciousness,
but I remain ravenous,
more so now than ever before,
for the words to cross my parted lips-
a decadent verbal chocolate of the
soul arching its way through minefields of disability,
letting go of what it can no longer become and rising
   again-
a phenix strengthening
weak channels of healing narrative,
a magic trick of flossing metaphors,
sedimenting permutations of my co-opted story over
fossilized priors as my courage quickens,
as we probe our way through darkness
to discover selves we have yet to encounter.

Because there is a wildly
unreasonable but remarkable part of me
that continues to fall into rapture with life,
no matter the outrageous price of endurance.

Gossamer

Svelte, frail and filmy cobwebs colliding into atmosphere,
butterflies' diaphanous wings—
translucent, insubstantial, raw mortality
close to flight, close to closure.

Gossamer—
the hemorrhage of my too fragile existence,

a life deprived of punctuation, of periods.

The arrhythmia of my world pulses with ellipses—
with run-on sentences running amok within parallel walls
   of my spirit
papered floor to ceiling with should-have-beens.

It is all too vulnerable—
this essence we assemble so readily plucked,
a piece of fruit not yet ripened, a dandelion not yet in
   bloom,
stutters to halt just when we are on the ledge of our
   unfolding,
darkness consuming light, exiling you from yourself.

Gossamer—
the rapid loss bated by feral trauma- the wildest beast of
   all—
the chance of everything that ever occurred,
plunging you into nothing save for a rotten husk.
Your spirit once an almost butterfly is now bottled
   lightning,
freedom caged, sunlight snuffed out by fear,
by the taught coil of pain lancing up from every surface.

I feel the urgent urge to release an unbridled primal and
   piercing scream at the unavoidable throb as life cascades
   into a cul-de-sac without affording me the opportunity
   to rotate the wheel, now fully outside the bounds of
   control, perhaps never within reach of human autonomy,
   to turn around. If only I could have bid farewell to my
   prior adaptation.

Gossamer—

you, or I, or the two of us, are landlocked inside of surplus
time and a paucity of space- the curse of trauma- this
monster without cause for the mind to grab hold of as
the body decomposes before adulthood saturated my
being.

I am an island just off the coast of maturity, slowly
reverting into disillusioned dependency of infancy.

Gossamer—

we are ripped wide open, our spirits skipping out of
us, rendering me inescapably hollow of everything I
thought cradled the world.

Gossamer—

I watch myself disappear, moths' wings surrendering to
torchlight.

I fear this game of hide and seek will never climax to
conclusion.

Tell me where to look next.

Gossamer—

my stoke of impoverished luck.

I plea into the vast valley of the universe to hear, just
once more, the smile in my voice begin to unfurl as the
resemblance between me—
this itinerant ghost lost in shadowlands—
and my previous self vacillates, double vision adrift at sea.

Gossamer—

the aggregate of dissolving selves brutally abbreviated,

souls abducted by the totalizing truth that we all pass by
ourselves, by each other, flying away to places the mind
   can never know no matter its intelligence quotient, that
   the ellipses of our parallel worlds can only be tracked
   by imagination, by wonder, fear capsized, if we slowly
   manage to let go of the human quest for permanency
   in the face of the ephemera that make us and break us
   into artistic collages of atoms dispersing through the
   inevitable landscape of time.

Welded

The bounty of life is invisible, indiscernible, indescribable,
arrived at through internal vision, a different type of seeing
more contingent on blindness than sight,
on the capacity to envision light within an echo of
   darkness.

This solemnity,
this solitude,
this shattering teetering on death,
this unexpected growth,
an evolving evolution,
this trauma and its repercussions-
a multitude of sorrows and intimations of revival are
   quantum,
evasive to the naked eye but ever so real and true.

We know more about ourselves than we can see,
than we will ever fathom because that type of vision
   escapes the world.

We must revolve our irises inward, peer into cataclysmic
  despair,
grope through shadows, ashes, a heap of fractured
  memories to fixate our gaze on our becoming, on the
  connective tissue of greenery taking root internally
we never before noticed.

This is where beginnings begin, where grief can be welded
  with spring,
birthing not what was but what will become, if we tend to
  it, if we water it,
if we do not neglect the path through the tumbleweeds of
  limbo and loss.

Beneath it all, there is a shallow footprint of beauty.

Can you glimpse it too?

An intact spinal cord does not necessarily equate to an
  intact life.

What do you think of my unformulated mathematics?

In my physical incompletion, I am questing not for health,
  not for a return key to the Elly in memory, but for chance
  to be with myself patiently as I am, to grant myself the
  grace to be more like water than a monolith, to let the
  hard swallow of my grief vacillate without harping on the
  gruesome and grueling debris because I have learned
  that this may be a vital pivot-point in my life.

I am still here.

Are you?

I do not believe fear can assail me more than it already has.

There is always more to lose.

There is always room for growth.

There will always be a lapse in language and
   understanding.

But I will soldier onwards, with you trekking alongside,
and through words because that is simply what I do.

Deluge

I am in pursuit of freedom,
or, in this scarce economy of dispossession,
scavenge but to sharpen an ode in homage to revered
   liberty—
inborn resources that should gracefully be mine between
the streak of birth and death,
ancient looping homespun rhythms
gliding out of grip for which I would splurge,
if only I reorder them from a catalogue.

You may be hard-pressed to locate the most
tenuous of threads yoking our realities,
save for the cyclical unflinching blind black hand of time.

The door to the ordinary—
scheduled appointments,
grocery shopping,
childrearing,
social engagements,

a first kiss kindling what I prefigure to be an ineffable
   feeling,
a lineup of careers and promotions,
and so many other mundane experiences to which I was
   not,
nor ever may be, privy—
was indelibly sealed by my stroke's blithe mallet.

For I have lost sensation on the entire right half of my form,
hearing in my right ear,
seeing in my right eye,
regulation of my temperature,
capacity to walk without staring my right leg in the eye
   and taunting it into mobility.

Thirst,
hunger,
scent,
how to properly prize out oxygen from atmosphere,
too many other absurd subconscious maneuvers of being
   human
sloshed away,
eliciting a cannon fire of impressions of once having been.

Homeostasis has unbuttoned itself into
a nonnative word sterilized with the alcohol
of reductive mechanism,
a pedantic exercise at a remove from my present,
a scientific anachronism,
now possessing narcotic appeal,
an antidote out of stock,
behind glass of biological antiquity—

a realm beyond my scope far off from my curated static of
  pain.

Oh, disloyal crucial aspects of me cast out of my reach.

Crawl back, even if your pace is glacier.

I have concluded that true trauma transpires when
you commit the complete English dictionary to memory,
yet the words you need to explain yourself have yet to be
  born.

A linguistic famine takes root in your soul,
carving the most massive canyons between you and
  others,
between you and yourself,
especially when language itself is your water, your
  medium.

You, reader, understand and you also
understand that you fail to understand.

Do not dismiss this cognitive dissonance.

Be in it with me,
this biting Prokofiev state of logic crashing against an
  impasse.

Oh, how I miss the swim of limbs
lapping through
bondage of hydrogen
and oxygen atoms
dancing.

It is only in this ill-revised version of being,
that I have realized the refuge in the thousand corridors

continually opening within fissures in my soul,
behind which millions of words wrap
their unyielding and abiding fists,
hounding me that they are not a mirror,
that they can neither offer self-explanation nor refraction,
but can serve as gateways through my darkness—
means of chiseling form out of formlessness,
offering me vistas into the extraordinary,
to letters snaking walkways through neurons that run
   through me unfiltered, a tap I can neither turn on nor
   off, words that beg on their knees for my soul to sing
   through the deluge of supreme sorrow.

Thaw

Disability not only transforms the body,
dismantling and disordering a once intimate landscape
into unfamiliar territory,
but also reconfigures time—
the arrowhead that once pressed us forwards
distorts into a distended kinked loop.
Disability lands you in permanent detention of the soul,
enshrouds you in inescapable presence,
topography of time emigrates from legible linearity into
   unending cycles
of now interrupted by stuttering stops that immobilize you
   into
marble as the rest of the world
continues to fold laundry,
contemplate first dates,
tend to gardens and purchase one

too many pairs of sneakers.
In our unfathomable version of life,
when our disrupted ring of time bumps up against
the unidirectional dart in the province of the well,
we cringe at our invisible war,
at our unworthiness,
at our drainage of time,
our preclusion from progress,
and at our sense of entanglement within time itself.
We are an unheard herd of spiritual warriors,
robustly reincarnating ourselves out of trenches of
    uncertainty,
out of storylines beyond our control.
We do not even know the plot, the characters we play
in the script, not ours to direct or to craft.
We hide from ourselves,
from the world,
from time itself,
which seem to discard us,
redact us,
trees dishearteningly removed from what was
deep entrenchment in undergrowth.
But we may be butterflies we fail to recognize,
growing ourselves within cocoons of skin and bones,
out of caterpillars of our dilapidated shells,
flirting with flux,
with flight,
with translucent technicolor,
praying that we may gradually surface from ruins into
    light,
into a reckoning with humanity-

our hauntingly beautiful ephemeral episode of existence,
our dissonance with others' aspirations to authorize and
    understand
what our suffering has illuminated is cosmically
    impossible.
For we have risen,
despite our feverish education on the cliffs
that being mortal means being vulnerable to our own
    powerlessness.
We have witnessed
fairness undone,
justice undress,
merit sullied
and endure in the tension of the petrifying but miraculous
    bones
that entropy occurs—
that a single step can alter, or even obliterate, an entire
    framework,
that our singular salvation rests in our unsung
adaptability to learn to let go,
to be with whatever is unfolding.
And it is just when my sense of
unworthiness erupts to occupy the net of mind
that I am met with the filled silence of a look into my
    welling eyes,
my mother's hand on my shoulder,
my father's unremitting giving.
I unexpectedly brim with thoughts that I am still
cherished, loved, seen in all of my segmented
    completion—
a paradoxical symbiosis that nudges open an

interior doorway I never before observed
welcoming the chance that something transcending
vocabulary thaws in boundless interiority.

Conclusion

The speaker seeks to reconcile the past with the present, her former body with her current body, and find a common ground
between them. She has discovered that there is power in her
disability, and she is trying to discover how best to wield it.

Movement VI
Duet

Introduction

Tidal waves of grief still overpower the speaker at times, forcing her into excruciating hindsight as she recalibrates her definitions of what she thought her life would be, looks through the metaphorical microscope at the way her life has broken open, and searches for beauty. The speaker is in limbo, both endangered and enchanted by her existence.

Radioactive

Atoms splitting, spitting out bits of self-
a fracture over which time does not calcify,
a break-up and away from our central scaffolds in
   exchange for platonic stability-
a theoretical potential that never arrives.

This life does not come with a warning label.
Our cells are not tagged with expiration dates discernible
   to us.

Radioactive—
we are all organisms and elements skittering through
   space, stuttering between no longer and not yet, forever

unstable, eternally mortal, always giving some of our
composition away, decaying at rates
dictated by the cosmos, radioactive since
the dawn of time long before the
Curies' 1898 discovery.

For nothing in this universe persists.

Radioactive—
patterns and congruence are but fluttering heartbeats of
the moment.

Draw breath and express here before it all passes.

Let's let our minds recede, our bodies intercede for an
inhale or three.

The leaves chafing in lambasting winds.
The swift flight of pigeons, a communion in transit.
The squirrel wicking its particular path perpendicular to
Earth up that bark.

What a phantasmagoria webbed into nature.

Make a shack in the now or hazard giving away more than
you can afford to lose.

Radioactive—
do not miss momentary marvels that refuse to leave marks
when the cosmos blinks.

Radioactive—
nothing is indivisible.

We endure only by hurling out fragments of self.

We live and die in a single inhale, passing like shadows.

All is under attack, on the cusp of fractionating.

Radioactive—
the tree is laughing or crying- who defines the difference?
Everything in this world is contingent upon how you see it
    before it blurs away.

Even these words leak feeling.

Radioactive—
the student in my inner vestibule—
that forerunner species of self
strained with too much intellect, perceived axioms as
    absolute truth.

But no body of proof will ever suffice.

This world is unintelligible, synapses into us and throws us
    away.

Radioactive—
too much scrutiny yields but heaping handfuls of not
    knowing.

That quantum physicist I once was prosecuted patterns at
    her
own peril of risking them, of abdicating herself.
She did not know that in probing too much, she would
    soon be forced to pay.

Her stroke to her brainstem ironically fuels my stroke of
    insight.

Radioactive—
there is always further to fall, a never-ending downward
    tumble.

I am concave, the world abruptly presses into me.
But I react by grounding through my sit bones,
exhaling into expansion.

This universe never catches us as we spiral into
kaleidoscopes of the infinite.

Just when you presume you cannot be decomposed
    further,
you must give more of yourself away, a persistent donation
    of molecules of self.

Radioactive—
just when the scientists of eons ago suspected they
    stumbled
on the smallest pieces of matter, on atoms, humanity
    gleaned—
through Thompson and Rutherford-
that these kernels of being were but amphitheaters of
    protons and electrons,
were but infinitesimal rooms filled with over 99 percent
empty space buzzing with electrons.

Radioactive—
there is no gymnastics of mind, no elixir to plumb
the incalculable, unreachable depths of infinity,
no Amrita, no theory of everything,
save for unrelenting uncertainties.

For the further you lean into the infinite swampy
    subatomic zoo,
too outsized for a single alphabet, or into shapes your
    brain
confabulates out of galaxies, you hazard offloading more
    of yourself-
becoming a victim of a radioactivity of mind-
mired in the infinitely small or in the infinitely massive,
surrendering more of yourself like the ancients frozen in
    the
metaphysical trappings of Zeno's paradox,
stuck in space you cannot reclaim
because everything bursts at its counterintuitive seams,
the entire universe untying its shoes,
leaving you spinning in a ceaseless hula hoop,
a jumble of consciously concussed subatomic
particles looking for static meaning in the world that is not
    there for you to reap.

Radioactive—
being human, shedding shells of self
we did not know we had until we didn't,
until disability ropes its way into you, an unwanted lifelong
    pregnancy,
weighing you down, stripping you down to bare skin and
    dysfunctional flesh.

Radioactive—
this stroke decays me more each day, encourages me to
    wonder
what will be up for cosmological auction next in my being,

leads me to mourn the feeling of feet striking solid ground.

Radioactive—
where do our lost hours, our decaying prospects, our
    continual cellular deaths,
our scattered electrons, go when they depart us?

Radioactive—
the awe and gruesome imponderables underpinning
    what it means to be human,
the tide of loss we cannot shirk, the knowledge that we
    must embrace our inescapable fate.

In befriending our own unmaking, our souls sprinkle new
    seeds,
growing us into ever-evolving creatures
that grieve and redeem ourselves into
whatever beings we can in this singular moment that we
    must
climb into before the arms of time swim away.

Beautiful ephemera

The crater between me and the physical world expansively
    erupts by the day—
its boundless dimensions,
its senseless seamlessness,
its enveloping enormity
encloses me in what feels like tense forearms around my
    selfhood fraught with fear
that I will only amount to an observant eye on this Earth,
forever ill-equipped to explore,
to feel tendrils of grass slick and stick between my toes.

I know not when this pit will become unbridgeable,
an agape mouth into which I will surrender against,
or, perhaps, in accordance with my will.

But maybe I will survive because my body will revive me
  against the opposing tug of my will,
because my body doggedly clutches at life, even when
  this entity I call me yearns to relent,
to let gravity sink me beneath the soil out of the turmoil of
  pain into eternal equanimity and
uninterrupted dreams untainted.

When was the magic extinguished from existence?

I believe the light begins to flicker in infancy when labels
  and words are ascribed to the universe-
when sunrise is subsumed into vocabulary instead of
  experience—
when the perfect concoction of incommunicable awe and
  bafflement
is abbreviated into something we call understanding.

I long to return not to my before,
not to my body as it was prior to this endless uprising,
but to my preverbal self-witness to the astonishment of
  nature
without ransacking the mind for explanations and syllables
that undeniably never impart the dazzling dart of the
  world as it punctures
your membranes into bewildering amazement
at the beautiful ephemera eclipsing everything.

This is where I want to find myself.

I will no longer engage in hide and seek,
in a game of tag, but I will find myself when I am not
  questing for myself.

I want to be in the happening, in the doing body that is
  one with nature,
not in the trappings of false understanding.

I will not find myself in the words, not in empty spaces
between them, not in pages of novels or mathematics
  textbooks
into which I peered for hours with the aim of making
  sense.

There is nothing to make sense of.

Senses are here to be felt, not to be fathomed.

But here I am in this body overcome with numbness,
  deprived of function.

For what is form in this world without function?

What is the body intended for if not for moving through
  the world?

I mourn my loss of rhythm, my heedless footfalls, my
  essence born through experience.

But maybe there is a new silent rhythm to be found in this
  disabled body.

But maybe I just need to learn to patiently listen to the
  muffled music of my body in this after.

Maybe the changing cadence will close the fiery ring
  between me and the world.

Maybe I will even learn to sway through the thicket of
  quiet,
hearing everything,
becoming passive in this wordless
empty receptive space pulsing
with being.

I will exhale here with the hope of finding balance,
with the gentle prayer of expanding while remaining
  rooted.

There is more happening here than I will ever know.

I am wordlessly honoring the rehappening through the
  tide of my breath.

At 29, I am finally revisiting speechlessness.

The light is hitting me in a different way,
its beams cascading through my entire body.

The grace of negative spaces

I once hunkered down over pages of mathematics
  textbooks,
spine contorted into parabolic focus,
drenching my unquenchable mind in
remediable solace of derivatives and integrals,
of multivariate polynomials I expanded or collapsed,
numerical and alphabetical accordions I played in
  accordance with my will.

I once kowtowed to the elegance of row reduced echelon
  form,

thinking I could contemplate my way into the vernacular
of the universe, mistaking our mathematical rigor for that
    of the cosmos,
for pages of truth written in indelible but invisible ink with
    stars across the night sky.

But, like these words,
mathematics is an imperfect art form,
a byproduct of ours not belonging to nature,
not anchored in the firmament nor engrafted onto that
    tree.

All of these languages we procreate,
fallaciously assuming we have uncovered the
bridegroom of veracity tattooed into the universe,
are distinct forms of formed waiting-
waiting for what I do not pretend to know.

But perhaps these formed forms of waiting-
for the words or the numbers to arrive-
are more bearable than pure silence-
that formless form,
that hammock of time suspended,
that typically breeds despondency if you are not prepared
    to marvel at your breath,
how it invigorates every corner of your being,
no matter how far your consciousness roves about.

Against the grain of my innate compass magnetized
    towards noise,
I have fallen into absurd love with empty quiet,
with observing the boundlessly fascinating humility of air
    flowing through my being.

There's so much to learn from the grace of negative
    spaces.

Let's probe these subtle molecules together.

How mellifluously they hum.

Can you hear them tango on tiptoe?

Perhaps this is strength hidden within the narrow corridors
    of disability.

Perhaps this is the inward growth that occurs when you hit
    the
carrying capacity of loss and aloneness I have in my
    stroke's epilogue.

All we do in this life perhaps is practice patience,
especially when our bodies have been mangled,
become excruciating tangles of flesh and bone that no
    longer belong to us,
that no longer feel or smell like home.

But it seems there is an existential derivative
yoked to universal happenstance,
an ironic mathematical jargon
engulfed in the entropy of what is.

However,
unlike in classrooms,
this derivative is forever gasping for a solution,
a looming equation only met by silent suffering.

Trauma never occurs in a vacuum.

Trauma is a vacuum,

corroding and eroding everything in its wake,
trampling upon lives we called our own,
disrupting ties that tethered us to our
very nectar of selfhood.

My mother,
from whom I am derived,
is the first derivative of my agonizing loss—
the enormity of death ripping through my life,
the grief that swarms through my bloodstream at the
   speed of light,
immolating me from within,
inoculating me with a toxic dose of my own mortality at
   age 29.

My physical form has been mutilated,
landing me in some perverse limbo between
being and not being,
rewiring the neurons in my central nervous system
so that they only come to recognize the left half of my
   being.

Tell me what it means to exist in
half of a body in a
whole world.

Has my soul-
that indescribably intangible vital organ of self,
too been tampered with?

Tell me, where does the soul live?

Does its geography even matter?

Does its location or its contours perhaps mutate when the
   body is besieged?

How does it adapt to fitful circumstance?

Does its circumference perhaps shrink in response?

My mother is physically unchanged relative to my before.

But she also has an after,
her soul disintegrating in tandem with my own,
captive to my captivity.

We feed off each other,
a cat chasing its own tail.

She is the first derivative of my trauma,
her valiant hardship multiplied by the exponent of my
   incalculable loss.

So, she may perhaps also be my path back towards
   something.

Towards what I do not know.

I do not need to know.

All I know is that if mathematics holds any authority, then
   it follows that if
I integrate the curve beneath my mother,
I may spy something skittering along an integral of myself.

So, I will cling to her.

So I will keep searching
for something whole within my dilapidated form

like this poem emerging complete from my irreconcilably
   broken body.

In the dawn of my life,
I am a shadow—
a ghost of someone I once knew intimately,
someone whose photographs I glare at in befuddlement,
a melding of undoing sorrow and utter confusion.

If only we could eradicate a subset of memory,
the dinosaurs trekking through our Mesozoic eras.

I crave a version of amnesia for the once iridescent blue of
   my eyes,
the dimples igniting the periphery of my face-splintering
   smile,
the zeal to be that once felt as a part of me as my own
   skin.

Yet I also thirst for another flavor of forgetting.

Until now, I did not realize that we have the power to
   remember our futures.

But the uncharted territory of time is often where the
   mind meanders.

In my mother's footpath,
I intended to derive and integrate a daughter in this world,
to cast the majestic spell of nature over her-
of wind coursing through wild wisps of hair,
of stars decongesting the terrifying darkness of night,
of daybreak beginning to break up the blackness in
   purples and oranges,
of trees letting go of leaves and flowers in fall,

of snow remaking the world into a bride dressed in white,
of the wordless disappointment of catastrophes colliding
   into
body and soul without caution,
of the miraculous audacity of the body's intractable
   tenacity to live,
to survive and to surmount,
even when the mind is met with what feels like
unbearable disquieting despair.

I yearned to demonstrate the pulchritudinous and
   petrifying
paradox of purpose,
how she may grow herself,
a plant in the desert,
out of whatever befalls her.

I would have taught her she will always have the
kind tide of her breath and the light within
that may occasionally blink out completely
but will always be hers to kindle so that she can burgeon
   over and again
as long as she is willing to seek what cannot be seen,
to listen to silence no one else can hear,
to pave a path at midnight that may be fogged by her
   own tears,
to let nature's unsung music ring through her being,
to recalibrate and revise the project of herself over and
   again.

Because if she can do all this,
I might have the strength to do so as well.

I will never let go of her,
this daughter,
this derivative of self,
who could have been,
should have been,
will always be someone entrenched in the
infinite causeway of my soul.

Holy grail

What is this crucial, escapably ill-defined,
feature we call meaning?

Perhaps it is the audacity to quest for redemption-
to inquire within while staring at unfathomable adversity.

Perhaps it is something within our genome,
encoded in a cipher we must decipher at the cost of
  failure.

Perhaps it is our Holy Grail—
our allegorical target forever out of reach,
the elusive ingredient that propels us forward
no matter how disarrayed the world,
no matter how shattered we become.

We extend our arms to their maximum span,
groping in darkness for the unattainable.

We adopt King Arthur and the Knights of the Round Table's
mission without knowing we are doing so.

We are simply being human—

mortal fragile creatures eroding under dictates of time and
   happenstance,
looking for something essentially immortal because
of our meek flimsiness on this Earth.

For whom would have thought that a girl on
the brink of womanhood could be struck
by a lightning bolt so profound that it left her in shambles,
plummeting the bottomless depths of a disastrous stroke.

No one thinks that will be me,
not until you are the one
turned inside out by the universe's heartless pendulum.

This is when the dirt thickens,
when the quest for the Holy Grail grips you by the bicep,
issuing an edict that now or never
is the time to begin,
or else your entire life, or what lingers, is at stake.

And even when your spinal cord-
your apparatus of direct communion with the sensory
   sphere-
is shorn and tattered,
when your brainstem is irrevocably damaged,
you embark on this endless, fruitless, search for meaning in
   dense silence.

Because when you have been slammed against the
   bottom,
when you are exiled and imprisoned in your own skin,
the only place you have left to look is within-
the one location the well amongst us never interrogate.

But hardship of this degree hardens you just enough to go
into the nooks and crannies buried within,
to breathe life into perseverance
you must muster to make it through another day,
another moment.

I have become so broken, so fragmented, that I am not
   sure
if I have become irredeemably afraid or undaunted.

For despite their antonym nature, it is challenging to
   disentangle them as they snake themselves about my
   being.

All you can do is keep breathing, is keep meandering
   for meaning, which you define and redefine, until you
   feel less breached than you actually are, until your
   unbecoming begins to taste like growth and renewal,
   until the absence of sensation on the right side of your
   spinal cord starts to feel like presence, until you realize
   your loss is a variety of death, but you are still decorously
   alive.

I want to live before I die.

I do not simply want to be alive.

I need a different type of strength to endure.

Tell me if you know what specimen of musculature I need.

Perhaps, together, we can shine flashlights on these walls
   until we eye its shadow.

I am looking, seeking, wading my way through

the waterlogged cavern of my psyche for all of the
  courage I can gather,
no matter how much filters through the spaces between
  my fingers like salt,
because there is a reason I am.

I just have to find it.

Can you help me?

Take me by my estranged right arm,
and let us kindle hope with our palms outstretched-
receptive to encounter everything we never presaged
  could happen.

We are human,
after all.

This is how everything always happens.

Endangered and enchanted

Descriptor of species at the precipice of extinction—
African forest elephants, Sunda Island tigers, Mountain
  gorillas, Black rhinos, our human souls.

We extinguish subdivisions of our own kingdom into
  precarity at an
outrageous clip, leveraging biodiversity heedlessly-
we behold the apparent inferiority of the beast, failing
  to see the wild spirit undulating under the surface of
  wildlife- mutilating our heritage, our bloodlines,
strangling our very selves, our capacity for altruism, for
  enchantment

thrust hazardously into endangerment.

Endangered—
we root ourselves to possessions that up co-opt us,
    consuming us into the ever-deeper waters of never
    enough moreness.

We crash out of self, skin unscathed, so we only know in
    hindsight,
when the physical floor crushes underfoot,
our bodily fracture lines a lens into interior dark shards
    lying in wait for us to assemble them.

Why do we thirst for so many belongings but are
    recalcitrant to belong to ourselves?

Endangered—
the immense library of the soul unperused.

The whole world is crying, its mouth juddering ajar.

Can you hear it?

Unclutter your ears with me.

Let's learn to listen hard.

Endangered—
we say too much, listen too little, do not permit questions
    to permeate lacunae in air,
meeting them hastily as though their disembodied selves
    were conflagrations.

What if we just let them hang, shirts drying in the breeze,
alone, unanswered, unmasticated?

Endangered—
we struggle to hold faith, dilate tension between the
    made and unmade world,
a rift growing into schism, as we make matter to matter
    out of opposable thumbs,
bisected brains, a burning blazing desire to colonize
    nature.

Why must we do this?

Endangered—
threads snagged over time, engines of us gathering steam,
mistaking uncreated nature for the proletariat class of
    world we rail, lash out against.

Oh, what a folly we make of ourselves as we unmake this
    planet,
hunting and burning it to a wan crust.

Endangered—
we are all radioactive, on the ledge of extinction,
not only the species we mine, miscalculate as disposable
    refuse,
but every organism winds and bends
through time, into disorder.

We compress faith under the hammer of entropy,
    crumbling and corroding sacredness.

Oh, callous and cruel calculations,
false dichotomies of the despot of mind, human hubris
    hurling through the planet,
writhing in our own disenchantment.

Endangered—
this game of go fish we play, giving ourselves away
unwittingly, unswervingly, not even cognizant we are
    playing until the cards
slip out of hands and trauma transports you to the only
    place left
for you- the infinity nested within your finitude.

Quit fidgeting.

This world is no stage set, no dollhouse, no rehearsed
    edgeless place.

The clock is devastated as we waste time- an endangered
    species of the now.

Why must you flee the prodrome of feeling,
symptoms of this life, side-effects of frustration?

We are being phased out of ourselves by the world we
    create.

Is there an insurance policy for the soul?

Endangered—
our souls are underground sewer rats- revolting, uncouth,
    unpossessed, unseen.

Endangered—
we will think our way, move our way, out of the crux of
    self-
this nuanced presence within—
we overwhelm with too much business, impervious and
    rigidly resistant to

just being in immobilized silence with ourselves.

There was always
just another math problem to solve,
another theorem to commit to rote memory,
another analytical paper on Proust to type,
an ever-quickening upsurge in the traffic of doing,
while dismissing the crux of existing.

Why are we so unsettled on the bookshelves of ourselves?

Numbers and letters whisper.

Can you hear their faint hum as they look back at you?

Examine them.

Examine everything.

Inhabit this body, this planet.

Let's go online within, not without.

Endangered—
our souls are conversing through the odyssey of language
    stretched to its limits,
the pivotal privacy arrayed in the white of this page-
corners for stray feelings uncatchable by black letters,
only countenanced by the exuded exhale,
mournful tears curdling to the fore from hollows in our
    eyes.

Enchanted—
this is where we hold hands—
in the chorus of unsayable emptiness, the orbiting
    dropped stitches

fizzling through everything, because we hold so much
    more than language.

The math never changes.

We always do.

Together, we thumb through a million and one
feelings that escape these verses,
that no vessel could ever contain.

Meaning lances up from
everything, everywhere.

You will encounter hurt in this world if you hold it in mind.
Let's let go of that leash together.

Endangered—
the acid rain of trauma, the tsunami of sadness,
the poisonous prickle of sorrow, of losing half of your body
    at 27—
the baseboard of the universe crackling into
a yawning womb of loss and the lost.
I bulge out of self, cut gruesomely out of my schoolgirl
    uniform at the precise moment of enchantment- of
    finding your soul unbroken, unbreakable.

Enchanted—
I disintegrate into my mother's hug,
entropy on pause, emptiness temporarily filled,
a feeling of walking on two feet I can once again feel,
a whiting out of mortality, a refugee, an alien in my body
    no longer.

Endangered—
in reality, I am growing endangered,
unlearning how to move by the singular slice of a needle.

Enchanted—
the shadow of my father's laughter—
I levitate, growing lighter,
as flimsy as thought without a backbone,
ephemeral levity ripping through me,
lightning, a shockwave, an unzipping of grief.

Foot-trails of what was snake through my brokennesses—
pathos for that Elly as deep as my once abundant faith in
    the cosmic scheme.

Endangered—
whether we like it or not, we all possess bodies, makeshift
    tenements in the world.

We are but clay constantly close
to endangerment,
to enchantment.

I lost my body,
but the heart of the world kept beating.

Endangered—
death,
a utopian GPS system, homes in on us all.

We all end up at the same destination.

Oh, intrusion of lamentations- interjections of penetrating
    cries permeate

my former presence, awaken her from the tin of memory,
permitting her to roam around in mind
700 miles away yet ever so intimate.

I glimpse her shrinking,
a pair of socks too often washed.

Enchanted—
she is still alive, a vanishing presence, awaiting me
in the vestibule of the universe.

I no longer fear death.

I no longer fear fear.

Do you?

Endangered and Enchanted—
it is not a trade I would ever agree to,
but circumstance does not care for human accord.
It decapitates you into another generation of self, if it does
   blot you out completely-
if your breath remembers you after it nearly forgets the
   shape of your name,
if your bladder and bowls unpause themselves,
if your body tells the universe it is still here, holding on,
even if you no longer feel half of you—
an internal seam stitched along the longitude of your
   body,
dividing you like mouse muscle fibers you expertly sliced
   in the laboratory
in preparation for the microscope.

Oh, this caustic collateral damage of a body at stake, under
   threat of endangerment,

boiling-over, back-bending out of alignment of self.

Enchanted—
no one can be in the present, as we each arrive here
   having traveled a particular path.

I have not rejected my history.

Her outline still shimmering within my present stitch of
   loss.

I have not forsaken her.

If anything, she is too tightly integrated into me.

I am endangered holding hands with enchantment,
refusing to let go, because being human
endows me with the remarkably inexplicable bravery to
   embody paradox,
an incarnate poem whose repository of words can only be
   felt, not understood.

Domesticated

You adulate me for severing ties with impulsivity,
as though the rabid leap from thought to action were a
   failure,
a shortcoming.

But perhaps this attribute was my gemstone,
my gateway to untrammeled passion,
to reckless bliss.

I had no time to spare because time
itself could not spare me

from its ever
quickening
cadence.

I moved forward through the world,
gliding on ice,
became my own arrow,
my own dart,
that landed, or at least seemed to land,
on the bull's-eye of experience.

But now, my pointed edge is blunt.

I exist more like a vapor, spreading in all directions,
or perhaps stalwartly stationary.
It is difficult,
if not impossible,
to distinguish the two.

Can you educate me in this distorted breed of alchemy?

The most ancestral segment of brain-
the crucible between my spinal cord and thoughts-
stamped by trauma,
unhooking me from myself,
a seatbelt not firmly secured in torrential downpour,
sidelining me from my world,
from my streak of impetuosity
that branded me into the person I was.

In its place,
patience sprouts new roots,
forcing me to waitlist living
yet still remain alive.

I yearn for my feckless nature to resume,
a video on perennial pause,
as though this stroke
a Shakespearian act and I but an actress
made up for the final act.

But there is no curtain ascending above the tragedy of my
    life.

I wait and wait and
wait some more.

This waiting—
the most grueling menace I have yet to meet.

Will you be uneasy with me?

Interference

This universe is not the network we prescribe it to be
    threaded thoroughly with the invisible yet presumed
    pinstripes of causality, not the fusion of one
Rube Goldberg machine to the next—
a cohesive comprehensive and comprehensible
    communion
braiding itself into an elegant axis of cause and effect,
a monument of reasons underpinning unreasonable
    questions that make and unmake us into beings forever
    fawning over logic, thinking the cosmos thought of it
    before
we loaded and goaded it into our submissive hands.

But this world was never ours, could never be allocated to any
    creature who breaks wide open and bleeds its way out.

This universe is our mother, our womb,
our tomb, our core conversational scaffold
between our inner world and the one beyond the
    boundary layer of moral skin.

Trauma jolts this central dialogue ajar, interrupts it and
    interferes with it so completely that our aim at self-
    renewal feels as though we are speaking across a
vast canyon in a foreign tongue.

For the totality of humanity consists of this single
    overlooked
exchange between these two worlds, which is distorted
    and garbled by
traumatic destruction and disjuncture.

We, the crippled, feel at least a planet away from ourselves,
from the world beyond us that continues to cycle through
    seasons
while we are ensnared in the trap of memory- frozen into
    a stagnant image of undoing fear, entombed in respiring
    disabled bodies.

How did this unhappening happen?

The should-have-been scientist, the almost
    mathematician, the near girlfriend,
is still bemused, is still rehearsing, refraining the same
    question, as though if the words became an echoing
    articulation I would be granted the justice of a response,
as though the construction of language properly
    constructed could close the causal loop I once, in my
    wretched, blessed innocence, thought encircled the
    stratosphere.

I feel so separate from the external world, from wind that
    whispers in a language my right side no longer feels.

What is the wind now saying from its distant shores, an
    ocean apart from the flesh and bones that once beamed
    at its blistering and enlivening embrace?

Reader, can you please translate its floating freestyle
    speech,
so I can chime in with you, with nature?

I am more at one with Dante, no matter the almost seven
    centuries between us,
than with my own peers
in his awakening "in a dark wood where the true way was
    wholly lost"

Even my shadow is interrupted, its contours blurred
    beyond recognition.

My very center and my very outlines have been muted,
    mutated,
contorted, diluted into nothing I know.

The universe unties my questions, proffering neither
    answers nor axioms,
save for dense dimensional silence—a blunt blade that
    cuts deep.

Can you offer me a bandage- a word or two?

I am a slurry of disappearing snowflakes.

Catch me on your tongue.

Legerdemain vanishes me from myself.

I see something longing to call itself hope in the firm
    anchor of a mountain
cradled in soil extending its extensive arms with fingers
    interdigitated heavenward,
perhaps begging for prayers to touch glimmering ears of
    constellations,
perhaps baffled in the same terrible awe and uncertainty
    as my finite, frail and beautiful self.

But, despite despair that laces my bloodstream-
an arsenic of the soul—
and feels like a boulder I try to fruitlessly swallow against,
I know right here, right now, something indiscernible,
    inscrutable and inarticulable is waiting for me on this
    empty and desolate white page filled with patient
    potential for the words to bleed out of my broken being
    into something approximating art,
or is it artifice?

Does such a distinction even matter if it gives me back a
    bit more of myself?

I do not pretend to come close to knowing anything
    anymore.
I crave only to become close to myself, to gather more of
    my felt self into my being.

All I will eternally know is the organic ricochet of breath
    against tendrils of my ribs, fueling me with a near-perfect
    dose of tenacity to transform my presence- to lift my
    chest skyward and emerge into something lighter than
    the dumbbells of loss-

a lever and pulley system that furrows me into myself until
I disintegrate into a cloistered secret.

Quickly, whisper me to your neighbor.

I will thank my disabled body over and again,
no matter how threadbare trauma's reincarnation.

Because, despite this unremitting unbecoming, my body
will never quit solving the problem my mind could never
resolve of sustaining the one terrifying yet miraculous life
my mind can only protect.

I will reach a hand through the boundless and bottomless
dark silence as I forge a
new frontier on this very page, meeting my despondency
to take the first step to encounter what I have thus far
refused to face,
to begin to let the dust of disappearance and disillusion
settle
so I can learn the new vocabulary of wind.

For in my desire to resume the conversation between the
ravished inner
world I carry and the world beyond,
I must start close in with the first step,
with you,
with wind.

Broken open

He broke a part of my brain
that put things together,

items regularly belonging within distinctive categories—
poetry and mathematics,
philosophy and art,
sublime beauty and chronic illness.
I have been decomposed
into bite-size
bits,
gone through
what feels like a haircut
of my entire being,
thrown against the drawing
board of reality,
my life spiraling into leaking
fresh wounds glistening with red.
The geometry of being smeared,
erased into a frenetic tumble
of discontinuous lines empty of direction.
I am coughing up assumptions—
fairness and meritocracy rupture into shallow
fallacious and flimsy constructs loaded with
    expectations—
that tear at the seams in the clenched face of trauma.
I am ravenous to begin at this end,
to be made into someone different,
someone with a modicum of power
over that which unspooled me,
compromised my spinal cord, my essence.
There is a part of me that destains
the ongoing ticking of the clock,
the impulsivity of cars to race on,
the neighbor but a door away

navigating the world—
gathering her children from school—
as though the universe remained
still and on its hinges,
unfazed by my upending injury
that shredded my existence,
a piece of paper into scraps
I will never again unite.
Doesn't she know that everything has terminated?
But I am still fighting for something,
however,
it is challenging,
if not impossible,
to enlist my will for a battle
whose trophy remains a
wide open question mark.
Time metastasizes into a peculiar
dimension,
cataclysmically punctuating my
after with post-apocalyptic
periods,
a ceaseless cliff of endings that
never ends.
Perhaps this is the only way to begin.
Perhaps this is the only way to define beginning.
I am but a fragile passenger
in the backseat of whatever life does to me.
I am not even sure if anyone
is driving the car,
if there is a car at all, in this desert of disrepair.
I am a body, existentially

and preciously confined,
yet courageously alive,
a bold splattering
paradox,
fragmented,
incredibly human.
I always was and will be until I am no longer.
But I still am-
a warrior frozen in prayer pose despite
writing god and prayer out of the script of my life.
I still furnish that control,
don't I?
I will maintain this position—
the left palm I can feel
kissing the right I cannot sense-
until the words begin their faint trickle into my soul,
beseeching something or someone in the universe to
    listen.
But maybe this desiccated silence
does not require hearing to be real.
Maybe I can hear it on the other side of my mind.
Maybe metaphysics can compensate for my dilapidated
    physical form.
Maybe I can mark everything I can neither feel nor control
    with the tide of
my breath, my link to the universe.

Perhaps its purpose rests
in an emptiness,
in the negative space that holds all of the lives sealed
    within.

Maybe I can adapt to what is.
Maybe.
Maybe I never will.
Maybe the attempt to do so will be sufficient.

Fixate me into this tranquility, into the sacred serene
    waters of Shavasana.

But do not lock the doors.

I desire to grow tendrils above immobility.

I will use my courage until I am whole-
neither restored
nor recovered,
but something
tripping on the approximate edge of unity.

I am learning to seek an opening in my grief so that it can
    no longer sink me beneath myself.

My limitations are teaching me how to strive for
    endurance as I exhale into
acceptance.

This spinal cord stroke,
a vaccine against the illusion of control,
is unteaching me all of the education
I studiously gulped down in classrooms
that I am the master architect of my life,
inoculating me with what now feels
like a hefty dose of venom,
so that I may commence in my after
not where I ended in my before,

but somewhere,
elsewhere.

I am becoming my own harness,
my own rope,
my own maker,
as I pull myself gently and gradually
above ground from some dark cavern.

I am surfacing into a survivor who grieves but who is also
learning to remember how to breathe new life into herself,
even into her unwound spinal column,
because she refuses to fall prey to what she is not.

Gravity

Our rootedness to the Earth, our entrenchment in flesh
  walls,
our zipping into ourselves by a steadying force, our
  overlooked
stability fastened to momentum.

Gravity—
our tenure on this planet is nested in the weighted
  custody of this downward tug on our being, this pressing
  undertow that is a brutal, indifferent, faceless, austere,
  yet humane educator as we fall, making eye contact with
  the floor, scabs scissoring across skin, blood gushing out
  of us, growing us up and out of the children we store in
  palaces of memory.

I have become a vessel spilling to the right, leaking out of
  myself,

onto the canvas of the world, a pitcher raining droplets
until it is depleted of fluid, an emptiness pregnant with
    potential—
gravity hijacked.

Gravity—
the massive heft of loss, the coma of trauma collapsing
    your
familiar form into boulders of sadness, a daunting finality
of the object you once knew intimately as a subject
    coming
to rest exactly when you were supposed to accelerate
towards the epitome of embodying the bold and
    wondrous
panoply of future scooped out with alacrity though
    mastery of
Newton's and Einstein's gravity—
that once upon a time velocity crashing against this
ruthless upheaval—the physics consumer darting through
    quantum
pictograms and equations, the poet drawing networks
    between electrons, concentration stenciling her
    countenance, spiraling to elevate corners of her eyes,
her dimples craters skirting her curiosity, the scientist
    betrothed to theorems, formulas, Occam's razor and
    beauty leashed to experimentation, that loiterer in
    bookshop corners, head buried inside pages of poetry,
    that budding girlfriend who should be engrossed in
    betrothals, not in betrayals, in childbearing,
not in barrenness—
now is a bloodline strangled,

a wire snapped between
me and
myself.

Come join me in my solitary orbit, in the mayhem of
 gravity defiled.

Oh, the gravity—
its doubling down on me, a punitive force that bends
around my name, corrupting it into something it is not,
the trauma pulling me underground into the alone terrible
 symmetry of a body I know no longer as I feel my face
 knit into bemusement,
my left-hand taking inventory of a right side.

Gravity—
how you swindle your way everywhere, corroborate
 your legitimacy over us exponentially, your underrated
 presence, your consummate effect, a cat we but glimpse
 as a silhouetted shadow of its aloft tail.

Hold on, world.

Keep spinning in the still motion through your axis as I let
 go.

Blink and a decade rolls by.

Gravity—
words tumble out of me, out of my right side, in heaving,
breathless expulsions, eager to leave a mark, the weighted
 weightlessness of black letters pouring through parted
 lips, the brutal necessity to be seen, to be heard.

Gravity—
the urgency to set my world back into balance with itself,
a crushing human need to matter.

Gravity—
the reality of physical facts, of gravity itself, discourages me
    now.

Your mind wants to win, to winnow the world as though it
    were a funnel, but your body is here to receive the entire
    universe.

Even my disabled body can realize unification in the space
    around me and within if I gently lift my chest and begin
    to kindle a smile at the opening-
the loophole in the gravitational black hole of my breaking
that has the power to transform my parts.

I long to know less, to feel more.

Are you overthinking yourself, chewing the cud of
    regurgitated thoughts?

Gravity—
the incredible desire to be illuminated, a fluorescent
    jellyfish jumping out of the sea.

Blink and years elapse, but the dark gravity of my stroke
    grows bone deep, reaching its sharp teeth into me,
    remaking me into a child bereft of innocence and
    wonder, loaded with gravity, with submergence in
    silence, hugged by stillness.

But now, for the first time,
I see the whole world from within the tinderbox of
  infirmity.

Gravity—
trauma tramples you into a Rorschach, a modern piece of
  art open to interpretation, corroding you into the brittle
  truth that you must begin again.

This is my start.

Gravity—
I long to redefine my relationship to you,
to the ground that once tethered me to myself,
so I can locate the unseen trove of treasures buried
  beneath dirt of my brokenness,
so human touch no longer tastes like fear,
so a loving hand feels like
a loving hand.

And it has taken me an unpaved road spanning almost
  two years since my world
was torn wide open to realize there is a way to feel light
  again-
that my diaphragm was and will always be my home
and my homecoming-
the trampoline nested within my body
I inflate with kinetic energy rippling through air
and empty with exhales bursting with potential of once
again filling, a vessel untarnished, untarnishable
by the indiscriminate white knuckles of chance.

Gravity—
you acknowledge me—

my disability not a pathology to be mended
but an identity that will, if we are fortunate,
come to headline us all as our bodies and minds
decline and decelerate,
even if life complies with best case scenario operating
    mode.

Excruciating hindsight

I remember a whirlpool of ringlets tickling the periphery of my face, sun leaking through the window, clutching my Raggedy Anne doll as though it were a souvenir from my dreams I could bring into waking hours.

I remember grits bearding my chin, melting butter drizzling down the top of my jean jumper.

I remember the thick dewy scent of freedom rippling through white and pink streamers fixed to the handlebars of my first bicycle, the wind whipping across my bare arms, and the feckless, unadulterated taste of fearlessness mixed with vanilla ice cream.

I remember gushing to-and-fro through the atmosphere on the swing canopied by the Memphis summer sky, my legs kicking me into near-perfect bliss and untrammeled smiles.

I remember biting my nails to the quick when at age 10, I found myself bedridden after fracturing my spine, the zipper of my innocence coming undone, the uncertainty of reality seeming to tap me on the shoulder and tell me it was there to stay for the duration and not having a ready reply.

I remember Richard Feynman dancing in black-and-white across a chalkboard projected onto my parents' ceiling, as I tried to make sense of subatomic particles, imposing the logic of the infinites-imal on macroscopic cosmic chaos and fluke circumstances, while adolescence and my connective tissue disease took me by the throat.

I remember strumming my right fingers across guitar strings, singing my way into my own poetry, generating sound over silence, and locating what felt like a porthole into my soul.

I remember running into lecture halls early, eager to select my own seat in advance, to crack open a novel prior to the lesson.

I remember coming thoroughly unwrapped like a malicious gift as my connective tissue disease locked me into myself—as bones dislocated in my feet, arms, and torso, as tendons tore and my neck grew unstable, incapable of holding my head on its once abiding pedestal.

I remember the hydrocephalus as it waterboarded me from within, filled my cranium with a surplus of fluid that doubled everything in my visual field, and left me capable of nothing save for sleep interrupted by the absurdity of chocolate chip cookies.

I remember my curtain call—what I thought was my final breath, as a doctor injected my cervical spine and promised stability but only handed me a devastating cervical cord and brain injury that outrun me every day, that unmake me by the day, that have caused me to realize the long gone blessing of simply having a chronic illness uncomplicated by tragic trauma.

I no longer remember what touch feels like, what water feels like, what temperature feels like, what anything tastes like, what any-thing smells like, what anything looks like on the right side of my body—which has severed ties with my central nervous system, becoming a decoy, an ornament, something for show that no longer tells me or my brain anything about where it is or even that it is.

I miss the memory of this side of my body, of this pivotal part of my being but I am unable to fashion and undress memories at my beck and call.

I want to cut out the memories of my past, pierce them with a fine blade, and place them in a box beneath my bed.

I want to forget because remembering is its own flavor of pain, its own kind of darkness, its own type of bleakness when your past no longer feels as though it belongs to you, when time itself feels as though it is taking you hostage, and you are at the mercy of every nightmare, every shade of black, you never could have anticipated.

Bittersweet

Despair hooks its sharp claws into your tender flesh when
    you absorb the
impaling shock of grief,
release your firm grasp of denial's motif you religiously
    rehearse,
when the remainder of the division
between the realized and the recalled self-aggregates,
swells to a volume impossible to shun,
when you have traveled through confined underground
tunnels of time and disappearance,

when your former self shrinks into an irrelevant artifact of
    delusion
and a different self you refuse to encounter routinely
    reveals itself
until you countenance the unreal and unfathomable pain
    and
devastation of the body stupefied by ousting trauma.

A different self is ploddingly unfolding from a surreal
    surrender of my armor,
as undoing disorders me, unsteadies me gradually and all
    at once.

You see, reader, you can die a thousand
and one death in the short span of this one lifetime,
multiverses of potentialities fermenting that fall short of
    becoming.

You select a path, or so you think, but the horizon before
    you quickly narrows into but a pinprick you must squint
    to see until the could-have-beens completely disappear,
    and you along with them, the future, the valleys of
    choice, desaturating into nothing but perplexing
    concepts that crack wide open, an interior set of Russian
    dolls.

This is outrage.

This is trauma.

This is the body and mind overhauled.

This is when the universe takes on Houdini's visage,
    vanishing you from yourself.

Poof, I am washed away by situations' bristling whims.

In singular moment, a needle threads a spinal cord stroke
    into me.
I melt into an aggrieved ghost amidst the living.

I am a shallow shadow of someone I once adored being.

I never knew I could slip ever so far away from myself.

This life is devastatingly fragile.

This life will break your mind a million times, while your
    heart sustains its steady
rhythm until it cannot.

I glance in the mirror for an eternal instant, starkly at a
    standstill with my own reflection, hauntingly curious
    about this person revealed yet unknown,
this face I am not yet ready to face.

What is freedom in the midst of a seismic subversion and
    sublimation of self?

What is time but the automaticity ticking of black handless
    arms intervening silence?

Was a clock born out of the atomic shower of the Big
    Bang?

Is the disabled self newly unwrapped a caged entity,
a slave unlinked to time and liberty,
fastened only to militant hardship and horrors?

The future and past taste like foreign languages,
rough outlines of notions I once knew intimately.

I was once cordially invited to interact with the world-
to blissfully fall into rapture with every gene network
    pathway,
every mathematics quandary,
each law of thermodynamics.

Now, my disabled body and sorrowful soul are guests to a
    different gathering
on another planet altogether, relegated to linger in only
    the singularity of this moment-
this inhale, this muttered word.

This is the terrible and terrifying mercy of my torturous
    trauma,
a crop we will one day all be forced to harvest in the
    hidden multiplicity of the cosmic dolling out of disbelief,
    disquiet, and dark disillusionment.

Except, I hope you, in contrast to me, are not met with
    your own evanescence,
with your own mortal eclipse at the beginning of
    beginning.

I would have exacted and extracted an extraordinary
    existence out of being-
the scientist in me was stepping her way into clarity,
my maternal instincts in transit,
my maturing independence nearly delivered,
my social world expanding in circumference,
almost implicating me into communal kinship.

But all has been confiscated—
an inescapable persistent blackout of the soul,

of the body waterboarded by trauma my mind may never
    be ready to acknowledge.

But, beneath the lattice of despair,
I believe there is yet a smidgen of scintillating stardust
watercoloring through my stroke's unmistakable stain.

In the dark night of my pain, my father hones the blade
    of his wit, and I am shaken by the uproar of laughter,
    especially when I discern it emanates from my being,
    something feral and free billowing up and out of my
    weeping body.

Revelation

An opening of a window woven shut by eyes untrained
to see beyond spinnerets casing its surface,
erasing splintering light, unthinking eyes
that only know Conrad's Heart of Darkness so can but see
    penetrating blackness
until their lids are ever so slowly, then suddenly peeled
    back,
eyeballs acclimating to unaccustomed light,
a foreign visual language in translation, a pilgrimage of the
    soul.

I am miles behind myself, my before—
the student clicking her way through reams of
    mathematical logic—
the keyboard an anatomical outgrowth, mellifluous rain of
    fingertips grazing keys-
the young adult newly furnished on the ledge of
    independence,

of maturation, of finding purchase in the yet uncharted
  land of friendship and romance, a mere breath away, but
  now
a breath not taken.

My former self is unfamiliar face that walks blithely by my
shadow in this desert of my after.

Revelation—
the draft in the walls of my soul, the wide-open hinges of
  my heart
reaching for memory through the medley
of cracked silences and despair slithering through arteries.

Revelation—
the existential throb of unanswered and unanswerable
  questions-
my stroke strangles Hegel's conviction that spiritual
wounds close without leaving a mark,
a scar.

Revelation—
Emerson's assertion that a life examined is the only form
  worth living tears at its
seams, bursting into catastrophic cacophony of
  uncertainty.

Too much meaning pierces through the silkscreen of
  being, breaking my soul
into smithereens, a fallen glass vase irreparably shattered.

Revelation—
please reveal less of this mortal fragility.

I have witnessed plenty—enough wisdom

born of heart-wrenching hardship to go around the world,
perhaps even twice.

I see the scrapes, the formation of scabs, across my
    essence,
as plain as bruises on bare skin.

Revelation—
I do not want to live this unlived life,
a coming to knowing the formidable opponent of
    existence,
the menace of unprocessed fear,
the smothering sadness of being torn asunder,
of no longer feeling familiar with oneself,
of no longer feeling anything on an entire half of a human
    body,
of feeling too human inside this mortal cage-
a blockade against experiences that should have been
accreting in the caldron of my spirit to
lease me some integrity, purpose beyond surviving.

Revelation—
the tragically beautiful realization that silence is an entire
    kingdom—
the beatific silence of breath fraught with emotion
    between verses of words,
the painful silence of the mind failing to make sense of
    suffering,
the dense fog of silence between me and my mother
as my breath almost left me behind,
the levity of rebounding silence between me and my
    father of soundless laughter at

the absurdity of callous circumstance,
the toxic nauseating silence of nightfall interdigitated with
    unshakable fear,
the three-dimensional silence that, against one's volition,
    becomes an exile,
evacuating you from yourself,
the language of silence my right side now speaks in the
    after of my stroke,
a book not yet transcribed into legibility—
this network of silent cities eternally
ungoverned and ungovernable.

Revelation—
the miraculous art of humanity to contend with physical
    disability,
desperately determined to see the light, be it real or
    imagined,
hiding within Conrad's *Heart of Darkness*, however
    minimalist and dim.

Because the human soul can compel the mind in any
    direction of its choosing.
Because no matter the tide of undoing, no matter how
    deep the well of tears,
I will always locate secluded rays of light in the dark,
caverns of silence whispering a music for which I am
    cultivating profound love.

Because here I am—
yearning to learn how to smile through it all.

Conclusion

The speaker achieves a newfound determination to focus on whatever elements of wonder she can find in the life she is living and in the power of language. She also begins to find ways in which her voice permits her to expand into the person she is becoming: someone who can balance looking towards the past with looking towards an uncertain future.

Movement VII
Potentiality

Introduction

The speaker's faith grows into a robust and unyielding ability to embody her new life with disability. She shifts her vulnerability into something no longer constructed of weakness but as a portal into receptivity—a reunification with her inner multitudes, a connection to her humanity, and a deepening strength.

Nested iterations

I am not an individual but a community—an unmetabolized heap of paper dolls that occasionally clasp each other's palms but, often, are discordant, an overwhelming gap residing between them. These white chains are bound up within the gates of my spirit where I endeavor, and frequently fail, to proffer welcoming shelter, to call them by my own name. How can they all be me— that untamed child with curls whipping in Tennessee wind who entrusted herself to the dirt as she gathered dandelions; that prepubescent girl who retained a capacious reservoir of innocence despite callous back braces and ovarian tumors; that ruthless young scientist who probed microscopes, investigating intricacies of proteins against the gush of setbacks elicited by her connective tissue disease; that zealously studious college student who fell asleep, cheek against pages of linear algebra textbooks; and this browbeaten and disabled iteration of that same person devoured by a spinal cord stroke? I had so many plans, agendas, and roadmaps into a future that only radiated light. But my signal fire guiding me—darts into a PhD, independence, a spouse, and perhaps even children—blinked into darkness, into shades of waking nightmare. I am sinking below the depths as time elapses. Can you descend alongside me, taking hold of my left hand? My life has become a mirage. Can you see me, beyond the scope of disability—under the surface of a wheelchair and tunneling tubes oxygenating my brain? I am looking for a refuge. I am looking for a look in your eyes, not pity but a filled sense that I am seen. I am rambling for a home, for that long-forgotten feeling of safety within my own skin. I once strove for so many worldly goals, but now, my bucket-list consists of a single entry: any awareness of any aspect of the right side of my body. I will take my pinky finger, even just the nailbed will do. I will take hearing in my right ear, and the taste of food in my right mouth. I will take anything and smile for the duration. I am a prisoner. I am the prison. My nervous system is landlocked in a quagmire of complete confusion, constantly notifying my brain that my body-plan ends at my spinal cord, my right side an optical illusion. All I want is to feel my mother's touch. All I want is to sit with the knowledge that I am on both sit bones. But I know I may be asking too much at this point, after 13 months have washed away, and my rations of hope have nearly zeroed out. The matrix of my psyche is irreducible. I teeter on a tremulous, fickle seesaw between skeletons of hope and paralyzing fear, lurching between extreme poles. I meditate, permitting the inhale to expand so that it can hold me in its firm grip and my breath can breathe me, but then, suddenly, I am overtaken with heart-wrenching disillusionment. I examine my latticework of paper dolls and the spaces between them, desperately yearning to tape them together so that they compose a strand, I can feel less piecemeal to myself, and I can begin to feel less tattered at my edges, less forsaken by myself. And I wonder, is this art project even possible? Do you have glue I can borrow, a stamp I can lease to timestamp my nested incarnations? Is this determination to rescue my past out of my disconsolate, perhaps permanent, present worthwhile? Who am I anymore? Who can I now grow into? What paper doll will join the ranks next? Please permit me to cut myself out into familiar shapes, so I can navigate this untrammeled, paranormal terrain of trauma, even if the only hand she has to hold is her own.

Defer to Dante

What happened to the restless fecklessness of gilded
   youth
rinsing effusively through my veins,
to my rhapsodic feet humming to the beatific blush of
   being,
to a feeling of kinship with everything electric roiling in
   chaos,
to a runaway desire for knowledge of particle physics,
mathematics, genetics and literature, to the blessed
   curiosity
furrowing the snug space between my brows in library
   carols,
to a spirit unclogged by vigilance,

to everything that seemed to fortify me in Teflon,
a synthetic second skin I could never, would never, shirk
    because it was so fortifying,
an essential vitamin animating my selfhood?

If Dante's assertions are valid,
I opt to focus my lens on his definition of 'dis,'
which to him means having traveled through a land
of shadows and reflection.

I loosen my overworked synapses to the Oxford English
    Dictionary.

Will you color outside prefigured verbal membranes with
    me?

This intangible fulcrum
in the word disability shuffles its
connotation from one chafing with
inability to one of earned ability.

We can spin a winter solstice into an equinox through
    articulation of undertone.

We, the disabled,
are inveterate humans-
we breed and gush survival.

I appeal to you, able-bodied readers,
to peel away from concepts as you conceive them,
to persist in undefined words that we can remake,
that can remake us.

If only we unbind the aperture of our tunnel vision into
    wide canyons,

feel the world churning as it dilates into boundlessness.

If this amorphous moniker serves as a suffix latched to our
   names,
underscore and italicize it with the subtext of superhero,
shape-shifting your intonation.

I am still paying my way into Dante's definition,
out of my own reckoning,
out of the trauma that acutely pierces me,
rendering even my mother's warm embrace
no longer a feeling of safety and security,
something to which my nervous system has grown coy.

Dante's notion,
while intellectually galvanizing,
has not made its way into my body,
a winter coat purchased several sizes too big,
demanding that I grow up into it.

This trauma is a time-traveler,
hauling me back-and-forth between past and present,
revisiting me in nightmares,
sending me heaving for breath,
coiling every muscle I can yet contract.

I am cultivating
a hearing in,
a being in,
a seeing in—
stewing myself in deep consideration of the
remarkably simple symptoms of being.

Loss procreates without end, a generative cycle of
  undoing.

Maybe I can learn to be with the loss, so it no longer
  consumes me.

But, for now,
each time I presume I unwind the final thread of my being,
fresh and unanticipated despair takes me hostage,
cutting across scarred-over skin,
my very body becoming an increasingly minuscule prison,
its shrinking dimensions suffocating.

Like a worm that bisects and
regenerates over and again,
this unfolding of the crux of my being,
of my body,
is at once a birth and a death,
my crib and my crypt.

And my mind, oh, my mind—
that cinematic rainfall,
that unflinching light,
that seemingly immortal smile—
has done a sort of somersault,
tumbling through a metaphysical abyss into something I
  know not,
into unaccustomed territory,
into an organ that now fumes with unshakable fear,
treacherous depression in the absolute alone kingdom.

I have never felt so at odds with this human form-
this person still alive but unable to live in the physical
  world,

this respiring organism who must,
at 29, redefine herself, recalibrate herself
with the certain uncertainty of what may happen next.

All I can do is be with the happening,
seep in now and inhale into it,
because otherwise my resistance will only beget itself in a
   vicious cycle
of further undoing,
because otherwise Dante's wisdom will never
infiltrate my neural networks,
because otherwise my mother's hug
will never again feel like my mother's hug.

So, I will be as I am in this body-mind complex I can
   neither feel nor control.

But there is an ironic freedom in letting go.

So, I will slacken the fist inside my mind,
to permit myself to grow like that bent tree bark towards
   the light,
however off-kilter,
however at a remove from the mainstream,
because here I am.

For even that slanted tree has the audacity to expand out
   from its askance center.

I suspect the strongest confluence occurs
when Earth converts minerals, water, sunlight and seed
into spectacular thrusts of color.

Will you accompany me out of balance?

Every point in space and within us has a center.

We just need to find it.

Or, maybe, we just need the courage to want to find it.

I will let nature be my teacher.

I will not lose myself more than I already have.

This trauma may have unmade me until now,
but I refuse to let it decompose me more
than it already has.

If this loss accretes,
I will let it appreciate.
If this trauma never terminates,
I will let it linger in my
shuddering bones.

But there will also be growth here,
because I am traveling through shadows
and am overwhelmed with reflection,
so all I can do now is earn the capacity to mount a
little faith, however ramshackle and godless it may be.

We are thwarted,
in flux,
reforming dim light into
tensile embers
buzzing with
moonlight.

We are usurped,
burdened,
breathtaking,

marvelous genuine contradictions
path-finding the immanent hamlet
of belonging.

Cultivating faith

In naming the world into a sea of syllables, we explicate and extrapolate into presumed captivity, we suspect we catch it in the impervious net of understanding, describing it at our discretion, labeling it into a semblance of liberty. But, oftentimes, this process is inverted, subverted—the infinite world naming us in our finitude, landing us in the land of objectivity, deceiving us into our denial of death, of our fledgling fleetingness, of how the ground underfoot may buckle at any moment, cracking us wide open, our personal rubble laid bare before our feet.

I have become the tragedy in this revised mutation I did not author, nor even deem within reach of my possible. Painstaking pain and trauma name us, claim their stake in our ground, exploding and erupting our entanglement in the connective tissue of our lives, dead-bolting us in the siloed singularity of the persistent present—an absence razor-sharp that it becomes untenable, intolerable, a landlocked scathing silence collecting life-size dimensions with white pages raked empty of words. I have been orphaned by faith, by the certainty underpinning classroom inculcation I subconsciously considered a fixed formula of reality, by my very center of self-conversing with the quiet vulnerability of being human—of coming comprehensively undone, stolen from myself, from time, by a stroke of a nanosecond.

In my after, I am fostered by horrific loss, pulled under the beleaguering tide of grief, swallowed by tears. We, the disabled, become questions we never before thought to ask, are stripped to skeletons and bleeding flesh, devolve discontinuous, diffuse from ourselves—our names become forgotten riffs, our memories morph from coordinates on smooth curves tending towards the infinite now into jarring stepwise functions that feel irreconcilably out of step with the unclaimed bodies we inhabit— fugitive faces squinting back at us in contorted confusion in mirrors, in the faces of others who concentrate us into a single thought—a dilute impression, a dot of pure inability. Please, have second and tenth thoughts about me. Give me back my multidimensionality. No further thoughts typically assimilate us into the whole people we are. We equal more than our wheelchairs, than our walkers and commodes, than our shuffling misalignment. Though hope I potted in my before perished, maybe its seedling has but detoured, contorted its contours in this crisis, a wound whose scab persistently weeps, draws blood anew.

Maybe there is hope I can yet rehabilitate or scavenge, even a single morsel of its yet undocumented configuration. I no longer need the absurdity of intrepid certainty, but I require a dose of imaginative possibility to ring through my remains so I can endure enduring.

We are on the run from our ruptured selves—
from dysfunctional bodies we never wanted,
from irreversible, callous accidents heedlessly breaking
    forth—
landmines across the incidental terrain of the world-

skinning us alive into our own ferocious divorce from the
  lives we embodied
until the narrative retaliated against us and our homes in
  the world,
forcing us to assume roles of observers in the bibliography
  of experience,
abstracting us away into surfeit abstract meaning.

If only I could donate some of my meaning to the impoverished well who know too much to listen to the unheard and see the unseeable nature of nature. We feel like the dust and ashes, the atoms, we all actually are. For, in our breaking unmaking, we grew inaudible and wordless—our wombs barren of what we once called apprehension, our throats choked by grief descending the wrong pipe. Trauma birthed us. Pain pierced us, thumbtacks on cork, into the here and now without any sign of an exit, a receding blazing sun surrendering to endless polar night.

Ironically, while I have become invisible in my wrenching unmaking—lost the irrecoverable slurry of firsts —I have clarified the invisible under the microscope of my internal sight, learning how to see inwards, how to grow myself anew from the inside out.

Why is it that the most exquisite and the most gruesome in this life are impervious to words, can but be met with a look of blended awe and terrible confusion? Language fails to fully form us; it is but a reductive formula, a narrow-minded economy, incapable of forming all the formless feeling—the beauty and the devastation that make us and unmake us.

I yearn to place the complete *Oxford English Dictionary*, even *Merriam-Webster* herself, on trial to hear all the words it cannot utter about inevitability, about immutable cruelty lancing up from the miasma of misfortune and the complexity of simply being alive. Perhaps we can pray—cultivating disorganized religions, creeds of our own making, tending to anything that reflects or refracts our truths with packets of faith, ample sunlight, seed, minerals, and vitamins—so these mechanisms of self-expression can ultimately cultivate us—hope, or do whatever it is we do when we are punched by our own powerlessness—our fruitless desire to build a bridge of vocabulary across the frightening silences in our lives. This emptiness we—crippled humans stamped with fragility—are encouraged to architect with new selves we risk not becoming at our own peril. This inner growth spurt bursting forth from trauma's iced-over winter into spring, this need to lean into the disquieting paradox of both rejecting our inherited selves born of memory and of giving birth to yet unknown selves who somehow possess our features in the after of life's brutal encounter. There is no meaning to find in this life, but there is always meaning to make. I curate mine in words, even as I am testimony to their ineptitude.

Disability encourages you to disarm yourself of the weapons of rage, grief, jealousy, longing, and loneliness with which you crave to repel onto the world, onto those who amble on towards romantic relationships, children, trips to France, washing the dishes, and attending weddings, and to take a step inwards into an entire country penetrable only through the raw credential of dislocation. This is there so that you can begin to locate ground to emerge anew into a survivor who wrenches open all assumptions about the universe that once stitched you together with lovely erroneous veracity—wisdom you never asked for but, nonetheless, received—the despairing present unwrapped by trauma. There are no answers, no finish line, no justice or fairness, no certainty, no mathematics of self, no reasons in this finite quilt of segmented solstices that crochet an existence. We will always grope for more and more that will never be granted. This life is a blessed undertaking. But we are still here with our ramshackle bodies, our contused souls.

Here we are—bleary-eyed survivors of the night that will forever haunt us but through which we can learn, if we do not relent to the onslaught of loss, to see dapples of light beginning to break though as we begin again. For that is precisely what the living do, what the living must do. I do not merely want to endure this existence—to be but a beating heart—for this brevity of being. I ache to live beside my disability, without waging unending wars against could-have and should-have-beens. I will try, fail, and try over and again until I am no longer waltzing gracefully between Earth and heaven.

Permeable

Vulnerable to passage of molecules, to ionic exchange,
cellular postcards written in letters with which our minds
   are not conversant,
a holding on interdigitated with a letting go,
the eclipsing evanescence of all creatures,
a tango with mortality,
a dynamic parade into and out of our membranes,
into and out of being, into and out of becoming,

into and out of time, always but a half step shy
from unsteadying illness, from an unpredictable,
  unleashing unbecoming.

We are porous organisms loosely roped into makeshift
  happening
with mazes of fluctuating flux, fragile snaking paths
  branching from spines.

Has there ever been a human lacking a spinal cord?

Permeable—
my inseam is permeated, a threshold violated, a synapse
  snipped.

I am a penumbra.

I am the night itself.

I am a hazy sepia paradox coming into view,
a reluctant recipient of the permeability of what it means
  to be human.

I am being born right here from the permeable womb of
this uncreated page weeping with unedited emotion.

Permeable—
I am someone at once so close and impossibly far afield,
a comet beheld only in the squinted eye of a telescope.

Permeable—
what happens to fugitive shafts of soul wrapped in a body
  distorted by disability?

Perhaps my right limbs are not wholly lost but horribly
  misplaced,

on loan from a library on Saturn,
fastened to an extraterrestrial body for the time being,
or forever.

Permeable—
oh, the waterfall of tears showering my cheeks,
as my right arm hides behind my back, baffling my brain,
my eyes scouring fruitlessly, retracing my limb's
    articulations to no avail.

Permeable—
even time trips- past permeating present, a palimpsest,
our nested dolls popping out of organization,
my inner infant suddenly desperate to be cradled in my
    mother's arms,
to be touched into the feeling that I am enough,
that this unilateral version of me blessed with sensation on
    the left side of my spine
is sufficient for love.

Permeable—
it takes me precisely an eternity plus seven minutes to
    locate my right ear,
now only ornamental.

Permeable—
give me back the innate, implicit, unspoken, once
    unassailable dialogue between me and my right side,
    once so accustomed to its changing position, to building
    temporary dwellings in space architected by channels
    now malfunctioning between my right extremities and
    my spine.

Give me back my pipette.

Give me back my lab coat.

Give me back my calculator, my once calculated world of
   physics.

Give me back the bookend of my body, so I know where I
   terminate and this spinning world begins, so the yarn of
   my being is no longer a tangled mess with the universe.

Oh, this beloved benchmark of my right side,
once so neatly packaged in the container of my skin.

Give me back all of me—everything, everywhere.

Permeable—
I do not demand with the aim of answers, but with the
   aimlessness of tasting the words as they percolate my
   tongue, seep into yours, so that what is no longer wields
   totalitarian autonomy to sink me beneath what remains.

Permeable—
on this page, I furnish liberty to do anything, without
   dispensation, without absolution.

Here, I am but someone searching the sky, finding shapes
   in shapeless clouds,
conjuring shifting forms out of formlessness.

This is my way to be with my ravaged body, my crushed
   soul, to come into the
moment with you as we forge a bridge, resonance of
   sliding syllables
permeable to connection.

Permeable—

we leapfrog along lily pads of words, photons ringing with
    meaning, an intangible but palpable telephone cord
    between my lips and your ears, the only two body parts
    truly longing for unity, teeming with texture of exquisite
    presence.

I have already been divested of too much self, my insight
    into my essence weakening, coffee diluted with surplus
    milk.

I refuse to become more insolvent of soul.
Because even though existence is fraught with
    indiscriminate suffering,
I am a warrior keenly aware of her permeability.

Permeable—
I am permeating out of myself.

Who am I anymore?

Who are you?

Must we know?

Can we know?

Permeable—
I am fermenting this new body, this undisclosed spirit out
    of fecund seedlings of self.

Together, let us let ourselves let go of the war waged
    against our wills, express the
yet unrealized signature in our souls we cage, set them
    free in the wilderness of disability.

Permeable—
we were always permeable to trauma, to falling wide-
    open into dark, desiccated restraints of infirmity.

Permeable—
we must imagine ourselves into existence.

This is how we become.
Eternity awaits me, you, within—the latent project of
    being human.

Permeable—
awaken before time retreats from your presence.

Attend to conversation with contradiction.
Linger with it without smothering it with fear.
For the mind cuts categories, shearing life into narrow
    binary alleys.

Permeable—
engender permeability to possibility, to vast landscapes of
    wonder.

My coup of self, a blaring alarm, a bleeping siren, ripped
    me wide-eyed.
I am finally, after nearly three decades on this Earth, awake.

Part of me is, intermittently, ironically, grateful for this
    crucifixion.
I wake to cultivating out of the cul-de-sac of tragedy.

Permeable—
I stretch interior networks beyond straight jackets of fact,
permeate every recess of self with potential.

Permeable—
all of nature permeates with endings.

But endings are eggshells breaking into beginning.

What happens when day uncrosses its legs,
stands up and departs into the insurgence of darkness?

Would this thought ever permeate my being without my
  stroke?

What happens to time?

Is it ever authorized to rest, to break like the dawn,
the sunrise, the moonlight, or is it simply always leeching
  wattage out of land, out of our bodies, permeating into
  heavens we cannot know?

Permeable—
perhaps we were planted here for these questions to
  permeate our consciousness—
to know nothing, save for the tender whisper of mountains
  across oceans,
the scent of spring tickling grass, wind thrashing through
  branches,
our own breath rising and falling with us or without us.

My brain injury thrusts me into conference with my breath,
a tendril I now always hold.

Permeable—
somethings, the overlooked, unheard discourse between
  our bodies and air,
we should not keep secreted too closely.

We must fully pay attention, encapsulate ourselves within
the splendid splendor of this moment and no more.

No more.

Permeable—
this world is entwined with stitches dropped, unbound,
my right side contoured into an imperfect globe.

Let us be permeable to beginnings, to rehearsing the
miraculous art project of innocence in the dense
spiderwebs of disability.

For even inside this pruned spinal column, I am still
permeable to everything.

Permeable—
soften with me into the temple of belonging, intentionally
listening to nature exhaling,
permeating us into purpose, into poise, into posture, into
grace,
into passageways we never before considered we
consecrate by reciprocating recognition.

Checkmate

Nighttime startles me into paroxysms of trepidation,
swarming monsters beneath my bed more vengeful at 29
than at age three.

My disability finds me anew in night,
kicking me around as though I were a soccer ball,
tossing my comatose right side out of slumber,

into frantic frenetic cellular seizures that ensnare me into
  the boxing ring of self,
popping ribs and extremities out of zip-codes of
  belonging,
my connective tissue disease conniving with my stroke.

I am a sculpture crumbling in twilight's twisted toolbox.

Interminable months expire since this trauma, but I have
  yet to adapt to the lockjaw of corrosive fear, or, maybe,
  acclamation to this degree of malicious liminality is
  impossible, beyond the scope of mortal enterprise.

The tears are unstoppable.

They glide and glisten through these words,
slicing the negative spaces between letters.

Even the firmament agrees, as evidenced by the sharp uncut fingernails of rainfall against windows. The entire galaxy, every proton, is mourning for something lost that cannot be replaced, enlisting some higher power—Einstein's cosmological constant, a steadying force—amid thermodynamics, an unremitting wrecking ball written into the world, winding through everything. My grief is a possession shared by anything and everything vibrating with vitality. I have absorbed a tremendous influx of trauma, a heady serving too overloaded, as though it were but a Thanksgiving dinner I could wordlessly and effortlessly masticate and metabolize. But it just dawdles, fraught indigestible fiber in my abdomen. Will you please take a turn dicing it for a while? My listless jaw deserves respite. I wonder how and when the word "trauma" came to headline only the ungraspable negative lived experiences, how language harbors potency to impeach us. There must be a way to uncoil our thoughts about this alphabetical strand, to unmake it and remake it, just as it does us. Perhaps one day, I can unveil traumatic joy, observe it flood my nervous system, mark it with a permanent pair of dimples. But, for now, trauma ropes itself around my bare feet, immobilizing me into crass vulnerability. I have hit a point of no return, and I massively miss the world.

Miles seem to accrue with minutes between me and myself, between me and life as I once knew it, especially as milestones strike—lightning bolts zapping me into bewildering disdain and disbelief at the intemperate thought that there are but two days between me and age 29. Yet, I am looking forward to bidding farewell to my 28th year on this planet, to the most terrifying ordeal I never could have imagined during which my future burnt to a crisp, and I committed myself, full throttle, to the howling abject task of enduring. So, despite commencing 29 as someone physically destructed—shoehorned out of my rhythmic pattern, indented beyond recognition—I am beginning, nonetheless, another year that could have not been. There is a lulling whisper of victory buried under this bleak midwinter. I somehow, sometimes, somewhat yet treasure this word—this redacted life—the bewailing document of my being a text in which every third word is ablated with red ink, transducing its robust scientific, epiphany-driven backbone into clattering illegibility.

But, I have yet to accomplish anything I yearned for in that blessed before Mendelssohn quartet, by this benchmark of time elapsing without me. Where is the first boyfriend? Where are the children I craved to raise, whose falls off bicycles and first affairs with vanilla ice cream I was eager to witness? That girl is laminated in time and space. I will aim, fall, and get up again to grow around her, ivy circumnavigating an amphitheater.

My trauma has its own legacy.

I do not want to view its imprint as a threat. I do not want it to hollow my breath, clench my muscles. The football fields between being and not being stretch by the day, and I wonder when the pit will become a vortex that will pull me under into liminal seas. I still desperately desire life. I throb to be in this world. But my body is at a stalemate, or, more aptly, at a checkmate, with being human.

Show me the pawns, the knights, the rooks, the squares of black and white, and I will outmaneuver myself a thousand times as the world bleeds time. But, alas, we do not come with manuals or pieces.

In the predawn, I am jerked alert. I glance, hastily shut my eyelids and then look again at my walker and wheelchair. The reverberating questions of who owns these accessibility items thunderclap through my mind until I realize they are metallic extensions of my own body—a fiasco of flesh and bone. Tears jog down my face, and I permit myself to decompose into moments of mourning.

Sometimes, life is too overcast with death.

I lament the inexpressible, the unapprehendable I fail to organize into language, even as I foist mine upon you. But, perhaps, the white spaces encircling my words will save me, will rescue you— sufficiently buoyant to clog voids syllables cannot, an emptiness concretizing with our emotion. I will never stop writing, because through these words, I am honing a sword against penetrating trauma. I will keep speaking my way into myself, distilling what remains, a vintage wine, even if it is but a trail of breadcrumbs trailing off, a shadow of a footprint or even a mirage. I am looking for white space between me and this pain. I need the water-wall of my tears to generate an invisible barrier between me and my once upon a time vision of myself. I am looking to be more inflated, more expansive, so that I can cut luminosity to heal.

These are tears of cleansing, not of annihilation. I am unintimidated by my grief. I will let the waterfall, so I am not stilted in a silo. I need to locate liberty wherever I can. It is a luxury item currently out of stock. Let me know if you can purchase it on my behalf. I am investing every cent I have left into accessing my own ache, so I can one day see something beyond it, so I can one day extend my neck skyward to see the sun kiss that patch of blue. I need to synchronize my present and past so that they can touch hands, however fleetingly, so that I no longer feel so static.

Maybe inducing my trauma out of its subterranean
depths before the looking glass is the only way through.
Through what I have yet to find out.
Let me know if you discern where we are heading. But for
now, I am bringing my tragedy articulated in my body
online and that feels like a feat of enormous courage. I
am determined to revive what I can. What I am incapable
of remaking and rewiring, I will store in attics of my
nervous system, because what once was something
I called myself continues on within, even if it is but a
subconscious haze.

So, I will mourn the girl I used to be,
but I refuse to forget her,
even if doing so rings me out in tears of devastation of a
   being, a life,
entombed in unwilting dandelion fields of my psyche.

Receptive

I recall the first time I sat with myself to meditate—the maddening silence, the blistering immobility, the holes where thoughts ached to intervene, the infinite space of awareness, the attempt to transform into a receptacle of sound, sense, and experience as it was in that very moment without striving to alter a single atom. It was futile then as a disjointed cacophony raged within, smothering the quilted quiet with a kaleidoscope of checklists and mathematics solutions I was stitching together inside my brain. I was unprepared to fail. Just being was insufficient, too paltry a task for my once seamless mind. I was not ready to temper my autopilot temperament. I was unaccustomed to being within the parameters of this very moment, this very breath, without peering my head over the barrier into a future I did not know at the time was only a future within the walls of this pristine present— a moment that will never again be as it is now. And I remember standing up from the meditation cushion and exasperatingly exiting the room, foolishly feeling superior to my fellow classmates for having "living" to do. Little did I know, I was the one short-changing the art of living, abandoning the contour of my breath, outthinking my way out of the need to simply be. And now, more than a decade later, there are no problems to solve that have definitive solutions. I am devoid of internal

chatter. Once the fragile link between brain and body was severed, silence became my music, my medium of choice, the sole
confidant who understands me. I am now more legible in the
pause between words, more grateful for the comma, the semico-
lon, the period, and the white spaces that permit me to breathe,
to feel comprehensible, and to become gentle and graceful with
myself inside a world and a body that misapprehend me over
and again. I now cherish the practice of meditation, of just being
with whatever is, expecting to fail, for my brain to leapfrog from
one fear to another but do not yield to the temptation to unwrap
myself from the arms of this very exhale. And it is not because I
have lost all else. It is not because the right side of my body is like
a phone that keeps ringing, a blaring loop of digital sound ricocheting off my interior, without any notice of my central nervous system. It is not because I feel like I am drowning, caught
beneath the undertow in the middle of the ocean as day creeks
into waking. It is not because I had to forsake a PhD in genetics
to relearn at age 29 how to walk again on a leg I no longer feel,
how to use the restroom, how to wash my own hands, and more
to the point, how to survive: my singular overwhelming occupation for the past 13 months that only continue to accumulate. It
is not because time feels all too slippery and elastic now. It is not
because I feel like a shop that has been robbed of all of its inventory. It is not even because my will to live dwindles—or, if I am
lucky, dawdles—by the day. It is simply because life has occurred,
hit a speed bump, a hard stop, and simply became a complex
undertaking. It is because failure filled my vernacular to the brim,
overflowing every aspect of my life, so I was no longer afraid to
fail, of just sitting with my breath flooding my rib cage and taking

the leap of courage to carve out a refuge within this very instant blanketed in serene silence, dark stillness, and solitude—my pillars of truth I will never again abandon.

Silence

I desire to be dipped in fresh spring dew, to empty
   pocketfuls of time
as I mentally meander through cracked, jagged side streets
   of citadels-
bastions impregnable to my disabled body, a
   deconstructing temple-
an instant capsized,
a moment eclipsed by fitful chance,
by the invisible infinite-sided dice of the universe,
the mercurial fiefdom of mortality.

Silence—
I lean against my historical rubble, overground excavation
   sites uprooted,
reach my gaze skyward towards the crumbling whole
   Colosseum,
stumble aimlessly down the Spanish Steps,
mingle with artists and artifacts in Montmartre,
listen to the whispering dead hum their doleful
   autobiographies in La Mère,
beseech the Devine of my childhood at the Western Wall
   to open the doors to his ears just once more.

Just once more, I beg, steeped in humility.

The price of this journey ostensibly contingent only upon
    the degree of dilation
of imagination, but the tolls are inescapably exorbitant,
the tax of my stroke exacting, lambasting.

Silence—
my feet, at age 29, can no longer carry me the places I rage
    to go-
adulthood a chapter without ending, without
    commencement.

Let me at least begin.

Ignite the flame of wonder anew in my soul.

Silence—
my ego is a fallen soldier in the warzone of my body.

The tone of the world changed, altering my looking, my
    hearing, my entire being.

Silence—
these words are too coarse to contain all I demand they
    do.

Life once held me and I held it with firm affection.

Silence—
but currently, we are strangers blind to each other, people
    straining to make
contact in stark darkness, in total night.
Silence—
all I hear now is a faint crackle, a piercing echo as my world
    contracts

into a pinprick of light, a gleaming, almost derisive
    counterpoint to my before—
my past superficial hurry through the miraculous
    humdrum of being
and becoming holding hands—
of the geneticist composing necklaces of nucleotides to
manipulate bacterial genomes,
of the frontier being forged with potential suitors,
of the girl who lived within the ordered entropy of piles of
science articles interspersed with Dostoyevsky.

But now, in this unauthorized after, being and becoming
    no longer lock eyes.

Silence—
I am under the leaden x-ray apron of three-dimensional
    silence stitched together with the mystery of not
    knowing a single thing—a divorce from foregrounding
    facts—
aside from the reality that a sublime uncertainty words
    cannot touch is my roommate in this deep ocean of
    quiet- a residence beneath my before.

I am gradually training myself to grip fear by the forearms,
to turn it around, to transform its shape into something
    like courage.

It will take me forever minus a minute.

But I have time.

Silence—
I have an abundant reserve of patience.

Silence—
I awaken in this thicket of silence with myself because
there is simply nowhere else left to go.

Silence—
the world receded, a tide from my feet, left me alone,
    behind,
a leaf shuddering, fluttering, trembling in riptide of wind.

I am heavy with a loss of innocence.

I have finally grown into my soul.

Silence—
there is nothing left to fear once you have been raked, a
    sharp fork skinning your flesh, of your essence.

I am a quickening heartbeat, a ribcage of breath, a
    throbbing absence of what could- have-been—the most
    penetrating wound of all—
arching towards the archaeological ruins of my soul,
eager to douse the fire of grief with spring rain,
propelling myself through grime and muck of disability,
to linger right here, to shower my spirit with as many
    blessings as possible
because I still am—
a survivor who should be underfoot with Ancient Rome
    but
who is, instead, dictating these very words, and the filled
    silences
between them, harnessing whatever beatitude comes her
    way.

Subtext

Spectators typically unsubscribe from my refraining
    humanity,
numbing themselves against the abrasive
discomfiture of my stark webbing into unfiltered
    entropy—
the unbearable stench of my disability,
eager to floss glances around and over me,
eyes determined to revert,
to rapidly exit my orbit,
to swing out of the lubricated bluntness of words
they exasperate to steadily tread-
a creaking syllabic bridge between us carved
into contortions of misunderstanding.

Incline into my transitional
neighborhood strewn
with wildflowers.

I am new here.

We always are—
disability is an accosting chill
hesitant to radiate warmth.

If life left you on my disquieting side of the transom,
never let me go,
even once the patient quiet spans spaces this poetry now
    dresses.

My dispossession is no spectator sport.

If you subsist on the fortunate slant of chance's skew,

permit me to possess you for a while, at least until my
   language tags the
admirable long fingers of silence.

Please do not bracket me between
the unthinkable and the yet unabsorbed
arrowhead of punishing potentiality.

I am more than a display,
more than a creature uncreated.

I hanker to sink my legs into weeping soil,
to drown myself in unedited nature in its gilded darkness,
its thorny roots winding their way to nowhere,
to perch myself like a bird on that baobab tree stormed of
   a branch or two,
to soak my soul in the Epsom salts of time and all of its
   tenses—
to be ravished,
held almost affectionately between the knees of now,
to be nuzzled beside every expired carbon atom,
to sow seeds of my becoming as they percolate against
   tips of my toes—
to feel dirt envelop my torso,
Earth fashioning herself into a permanent skirt.

I hunger to return to something primordial,
even if that means I am an aimless sea of quarks and
   neutrinos,
puddles of particles without direction or velocity.

For this ever-breaking body is already
homeless of form and proportion,
already has nothing to left to lose.

Will you hazard everything you no longer have with me?

The entire tent of my essence collapsed,
the integral of my previous 29 years
but a sentence preceding a painful period.

However, unlike grammar, my life catapulted into an
unmaking depleted of the beauty of word selection or
  premeditation.

Toss me a thought to chew and chew,
and I will live a little inside your thought.

I am not sure how to be here—
how to sufficiently thicken my skin so it becomes
rough like the burnt sienna bark of that tree,
how to become me inside this body unprimed for this
  adaptation.

I am 29, but my indented physicality is ever so estranged
  from this age.

Do you feel the number time etches onto you?

Can we begin from where we feel we are?

And my spirit—
or whatever intangible aspect we call the self—
in this aftermath has aged a millennium in just a year and
  change.

I am ancient where it counts.

Do you know how to count what counts?

Has the word shaken you upside down yet with that terse
unapologetic mathematical lesson?

I am soil ill-defined and unbound.

Perhaps that is precisely where home penetrates us all:
in the sublime subtext of landscapes tapering just out of
    sight.

But aren't we always petering just out of our own
    periphery?

Isn't that exactly where we are found?

Lacunae

Emptiness borne of the erosion of time, blotting out text in
    ancient manuscripts,
fissures in skeletons, pits of discontinuity, overwintering
    trauma's self-erasure, vulnerable points of access, fault
    lines demarcating what it means to be mortal,
unfilled and unfillable cosmic cavities that mute and
    mutate us.

This revised, redacted life-
my crestfallen creature-hood entombed in planetary
    lacunae,
constrained in a dark hole in a confined corner,
unseen,
unheard,
unlived.

Lacunae—
are you my newfound concavity
of hope, of courage?

Lacunae—
you are my salvation, the tendon on which I offload myself,

gradually emigrating up and out from beneath plodding
   footfalls of
undoing loss piggybacking on permanent irrelevance of
   swift tragedy,
dragging landslides of weighted feeling,
an endless haptic feedback loop, a doubling down of
   gravity.

Lacunae—
we are always overpowered by this inherited human
   wound.

What happened to the once unworried, intentional,
   unfurrowed space between my
eyebrows, the wispy kite of my being in flight everywhere?

Lacunae—
a critical uneasy vacancy, a respiring ghost concealed
   beneath skin.

Lacunae—
a resolute danger zone, uncharted, indubitable, fastidious.

I exist in nightmares unimagined.

Why would you concoct this reality in mind when you
   watercolored oceans in cerulean, solved unassigned
   linear algebra problems out of infatuation with the
   poetics of matrices, when you felt glee swipe across your
   face as you remedied faulty recombination between
   pairs of DNA ribbons, when you pipetted culices of
   genomes into neat stacks of tubes, when the world
   appeared as an intact discernible textbook, depleted of
   lacunae,

flipped open to the exact page calling your attention,
when everything was in supposed-to-be configuration,
not a cabal, a nauseating stack of betrayals and blessings,
when a stroke was outside the bounds of your thoughts,
not a single staggering millisecond misplaced?

Lacunae—
sincere ambassadors of who we are.

Lacunae—
I am rebranded by you.

I go looking for my former self, a code stitched into my
    memory, accessible in the
seething dark lacunae of dreams.

The shingles of my roof—attacked, irreparable, wailing
    with lacunae.

Lacunae—
I am behind my own schedule,
a local bus slogging along in slumber, ontological
    lassitude.

Lacunae—
I exist in some inner annex, marked with abject lacunae,
    prison tattoos,
compostable in my wheelchair.

I am a jungle of recycled parts not intended for juncture,
the lacunae in the highway of my spine,
the weeping leaking of my right half,
oozing droplets of spatial acuity, a searing sharp cry
of silence tumbling through the annals of my spilling
    body.

I am quietly enclosed in the parentheses of disability,
now a footnote in the trampled text of my physicality-
this document reeling, striving to breathe.

Lacunae—
the vagaries of the world that dent us all.

Lacunae—
the portal of my right side pulling its way into my left,
two masses of land shifting across a vast sea,
merging articulations of strangers barricaded by strange
    languages.

When I interlace my fingers, my left-hand landing on an
    unknown bedfellow,
my right hand—hollow, numb, a living monument of
    lacunae.

I issue myself edicts soundlessly as I bemoan the darkness,
faltering to witness pale interior light gathering
poise, grace, integrity, the unaccustomed virtue of lush
    interior authenticity budding through the hours.

Lacunae-
terrain of the unknown—
does the future have a birth date?

The drizzle of meaning cementing into words untangling
    their way out of lamentation's soundscape blended with
    the thrum of
oxygen concentrators swelling with tears.

What happens to my words when they become you?

Lacunae—
entropy of tumbling tenses in turmoil, under tension of
    our expectations.

The shadow of my ultrasound as a fetus overlapped by the
    shadow of my existence, now fluttering.

Lacunae—
what does a book feel at boundary-crossing moments as
    we trespass its
organless, senseless,
parched parchment skin?

Lacunae—
shared hollow fistulas between us and books.

Books rely on me, on you, to embody them out of their
    tombs.

Lacunae—

I am too brimming with you, too akin to inhuman books,
    desperately desiring not to evoke, but to feel, love—
to be caressed, kissed, cherished by mortality, not by
    eternal pages.

Lacunae—
it has taken me three decades to hear molecules in air, to
    see them without hankering to know them, to smile at
    what I do not fathom, at the marvel of the gears
endlessly rolling through this unknowable world tethered
    with lacunae.

My right fingers tickle the air, lacunae of piano keys packed
    with nitrogen and oxygen.

My right-hand quivers with sublime music
unheard, unhearable, raw and real.

Lacunae—
we are elusive, blurred beings circumnavigating the
  general zip code of self but skipping over our own
  interiority, eclipsing our own souls.

If only we could just be without carrying the ostensibly
  crucial cloak of enterprising accomplishment and
  resumes.

Lacunae—
I stirred into waking—
as anesthesia left my bedside, my soul walked into my
  being just as my right leg forgot how to walk.

Lacunae—
99 percent of the body lives in silence.

Can you cope with the lacunae you cannot seal over with
  stuffing?

Can you sit with them with me?

Lacunae—
Earth migrates 18 miles each second around the sun.
But I can be still here, at a semblance of rest with and
  residence within lacunae.

Be here with me.

Lacunae—
we rely on you.

Some facts are best left to themselves.

You, as I did, distort awareness into a funnel—questing
    to isolate mechanistic rudiments of that gene
    network pathway at the price of the remainder of the
    stratosphere.

Lacunae—
let's define awareness as the complete totality of the now
    happening,
unfolding like these words as they descend on your ear,
    my tongue.

I will take this ragged body and fuller moon of a soul over
    that full-toothed body and the ghostly shell of a soul I
    never knew dwelled within.

Lacunae—
I wish being human gave us a vote, but fate finds us.

Lacunae—
let's exhale into the grip of lacunae.

We can even sing into the bottomless, embodied
divorce of happenstance, because in these lived lacunae,
    we meander from being in our own neighborhood into
    the clarity of our essential essence,
the lacunae lingering at the bleeding
beating heart of being human.

Surfacing

You may assert that my life has been curtailed,
that life has happened to me—
has ripped away the floor beneath my feet,
has caved in the roof overhead,

has brought me so intimately close to grief that I am now
  holding hands
with death as I linger on Earth,
has modeled me into the paragon of sorrow.

But I will tell you differently.

My existence may fall within the classification of science
  fiction due to the disjuncture between the right side
  and my brain, due to deafness in my right ear, due to
  my hijacked visual landscape, due to my impoverished
  oxygen levels and a ceaseless list that is not the
  heartbeat of this poem.

I will tell you that when my ceiling collapsed- when
  I leapfrogged from pursuing a PhD to becoming a
  scientific marvel of my own—the sky still held me up.

When the bottom underfoot gave way, my soul rerouted
  itself, discovering that the absence of anything in my
  right leg did not translate to immobility, but rather to
  fashioning my own wings out of the depths of dazzling
  despair.

In this grief,
a book that never ends no matter how often you pick it up,
there is a gentle elegance.

I search with a flashlight for mourning,
but it has stood up,
transported itself out of me,
out of my undesigned body—
so long a watershed of self-reproach.

Can you see me flickering, a dimple of translucent light?

I am a sculpture,
stilled along a purposeful path,
sunken out of contact.

But now, I have you.

Touch me, please, so I dilate alive.

Finally, at the synapse between us, I am surfacing.

I thought that in coming so close,
in looking at my trauma and sadness in the eye,
I would either bolt in some other direction,
or it would somehow slaughter me from within.

But, in the passage of 13 months,
I have run out of places to run.

I have yet to blink.

At age 29, all I have come closer to in examining the
   breadth of my stroke,
is a oneness with the knowledge that we are all mortal,
that everything passes transiently through this beautifully
   bleak planet.

I no longer fear my own death but view it as an invitation
   to live fully and candidly,
even if that life is not the life I intended.

Whom among us truly succeeds in this endeavor?

I have found a field of joy in this untamable sorrow.

When my very breath was called into question,

I almost had to let go.

Now that I know that the letting go will come, my hunger to hold on has only ossified into something immortal at the bottom of the ocean.

Stitches dropped

Swallowed by morasses of knowledge, we find ourselves lost in numerical abstraction, decomposing our atomic composites into a manifold of myopic polynomials, giving ourselves away in exchange for hasty summations, for superficial solutions, for proofs followed by QED, as though a Latin acronym could be the period at the end of the unending cosmos. We pay the exorbitant price of the unspeakable profundity raining through nature, through ourselves.

We only learn in our own unmaking,
in the body's inevitable reverse engineering,
that no erudition will ever equal the awe swelling
in the eyes of the unschooled child you once were at the
    multitude of the miraculous
irreducible to strings of numbers and letters,
to the simplicity of a complex theorem.
Why must we understand so much?
Perhaps I know too much.
Perhaps I know too little.
Do you need to calculate the kinematics of the dove's fight
    to gawp at its
perfect poetic perplexity?

Does not the innocence born of a lack of such knowledge
render it all the more thickened with magic, with
amazement and a zeal to be so fully alive, so blown by
icy gusts disarraying curls, the frost curdling its way into
the bones of your soul that you cannot help but smile
in midstream of being a creature- so feeble, frail, yet
unabashedly here—this soft half-moon of flesh that is
here but a moment.

But a moment.
Hold on.
Be ready to let it all go.
For there is no way to tabulate infinity, perhaps only a
secret harvested in the soul.
Do you still need proof, axioms or theorems?
Do I?

Do we still need calculations to witness the magisterial
landscape of stars' choreography, to be within the
whispering hum of the simultaneity of dazzlement and
loss as we disappear ourselves into their celestial sprinkle
through the darkness?
We are one with the light finding a home in night
overhead-
embers riding through time and space,
atoms gaining mass and momentum
rung through with consciousness,
with selves we call 'I.'

How can we begin to apprehend the emergence of this
'I'out of subatomic particles weaving us
into being through time? For people are not polynomials,
do not come with manuals, with abstruse academia

we seek to solidify into what we call sense in this brief
band of time. There is nothing here to fear, not anymore
anyways, not after a stroke stuck me down,
lightning slammed
against metal.
We are born with holes,
with stitches dropped.

There is nothing here to fathom. Of course, certain truths,
conservation of energy, may filter through this world but
others, the bottomless, indecipherable and surreal reality
of the soul, are impossible to pin down, to manipulate
with a calculator. Try and you will fail. I am only preaching
this irrefutable veracity because I endeavored, because I
was in your shoes—
a manifest scientist eager to settle physics, math and
human biology into the rigid rigor of equations,
a human who shrugged off notions of mortality
like unwarranted layers of clothing in sweltering summers
in her quest to figure things out, to amass too much
understanding that she nearly unwittingly drowned in its
depths as she migrated further from the shore of being
incurably human.

But she blinked her eyes and blew away, a single solitary
thrashing wind swiping her of all that was, of all that
could have been her, my, life. She and I are both still in
disbelief, thunder still finding us long after the storm?

Precisely when we are most vulnerable—when our hinges
break, when we need to be held in all of our fractured
humanity on the island of infirmity that curses and

blesses us with far too much time and far too limited space—we are stripped to statistics, to numbers whose contours are too callous, too calculating, too unbearably scientifically reductive for our broken bodies that we begin to retaliate against this overly medicalized reaction by ever so slowly, unbeknownst to ourselves, returning to the shorelines of the children we were and still carry within- learning, against our wills, that as the body crumbles, the soul somehow remains unscathed, its roots only deepening as it undergoes a growth spurt, enriching us, germinating us from within.

This body is an irreparable deluge of pain, a malaise of pieces that dislocate on the right half of me I no longer sense- my injury splitting me, a piece of bread neatly bisected, down my axis of symmetry, stealing an entire two quadrants of my once magnificent whole.
But there is something happening within, incalculable, ineffable.
There is a soul spinning spinneret of golden light out of the darkness,
an eternal luminosity no devastating upheaval of a life can snuff out
fully as these verses crawl out of my interior,
tulips blooming out of the patience I grew into
as my trauma taught me that I could be my
own belonging,
sunrise painfully unfolding from
a silhouetted eclipse,
that if I do not resist this friction-filled

version of life, the world can be as it was when I was a
  head-full
of undying curlicues skipping through
tall grasses soaked with sunlight—
something boldly burgeoning out of stardust,
collapsing and rising like the river,
letting myself let go and be swept away by the cryptic
  crucible of nature untrammeled by too much knowing.
I will find the peaks in this dark life I neither authored nor
  sanctioned.
I will find the magic without the microscope,
eschewing the focus that undoes the beauty of this world.
Oh, these words—how they overfill my interior with
  wonder.
In their midst, I weld myself into a witness, a defiant
  survivor, the one who still
brazenly extends her neck skyward to see the internal sky
  from her post in her sickroom—her prison and my ticket
  to liberty.

Syllables

Monomers beaded into words, coverlets of meaning,
  invisible networks of articulation between brains, the
  communion binding spirits, routes of escape into
  alternative worlds percolating on pages, rivers of quanta,
  of luminosity, searching for belonging in sentences.

We all seek home in the crook of an elbow, the warmth of
  a maternal embrace,

the strength of paternal shoulders, an unspoken, unheard
   exchange between knowing eyes, in our bodies,
   however ornery and disabled,
in musical octaves, poetry and prose, in ephemeral
   eternity.

Syllables—
my world has altered its shape, bruised its boundaries,
   confounding my sense of place.

I am not afraid of the teetering precipice of trauma
because right here, I have nothing left to lose, everything
   to gain.

Syllables—
my impoverished sensation is a blitzkrieg out of context of
   a world war, trauma
morphing me beyond my body as I first met it, recalling
   me
like an item out of date, out of stock, emptied of purpose.

Syllables—
what a decadent stroke of fortune.

Syllables—
flashlights into all that has been dismembered.

Cloudy, starlit, winged creatures so celestially fleeting, so
   uncatchable,
so infinitely subatomic.

Syllables—
trauma undoes the virtue of certain syllables, forces them
   to amass too much mass,

perforating the connective sheath of my soul, a canyon
  overflowing with scorching lava, incisive daggers that
  lodge somewhere between my sternum and trachea,
  furrow their way into the dark pit of my stomach.

Syllables—

a disarming disavowal, an emigration of words once
  glazed with love out of my body into abstraction, a rush
  of syllables nicked of embodiment.

I have witnessed the brutality of
mathematics unmade,
science unmade,
my becoming unmade,
my being unmade.

Syllables—

an evocative echo of mass shooting of rules and
  regulations, of logic and coherency.

I am the victim.

I am the survivor.

Syllables—

the word walk is not merely a trigger but a perpetually
  loaded
gun pointing into the interior of my soul.

What happened to beauty and integrity?

Where did their outlines metastasize?

Syllables—

the necklace that shatters against the vehemence of
  trauma—days, time, the calendar

falling away, scraping their palms, into irrelevant
   surrealism.

The cruel curse of being human is that we are all broken,
   breaking, or breakable—
a truth indifferent to our retaliation and retort.

Syllables—
the immortality of our dreamscape nested within waking
   mortal nightmares.

For we are no glass sculptures that rupture out of shape
   into shards.

We break but, somehow, remain human, our smithereens
   of selves
canistered in our interiors.

Syllables—
I view this blank page as an essential opportunity to rebel,
   to do something
outrageously iconoclastic, to break the mold of form and
   structure, to undo the word's
expectations in recompense for its undoing of me.

Syllables—
sometimes, I need to fracture the bones of syllables, to
   surround myself in sublime silence—the only mercy
   in the riptide of my now—to hear the invincible,
   indefatigable
symphony of breath hitting the howling landscape of my
   body, to see only
with eyelids shut a blazing blue sky crackling with robins,
   to let myself

let go of duffle bags overcome with bricks of trauma, loss
 and disability.

Syllables—
I need you, my sheer infatuation and magnetization to
 your majesty.

But, sometimes, I also need to leave myself alone in
 unspeakable moments of being,
to set you free so that I can ever so hesitantly learn to
 be patient and gentle with this body I despise, so that
 syllables are stripped away from this heartbreaking
story of the right half of my body, so that I can overwrite
 this
eulogy into a placid song.

It will take time, but I have a warehouse of patience.

Syllables—
please wait for me to find you in prayer, in hope, in the
 once upon-a-time
rightness of my right side.

Harmonic

In the wake of trauma, self-sabotage hounds the why question—
a pernicious echo of emptiness gushing between reality and the
storyline of how we expected our lives to unfold, as if life were
something one could order off a menu. But this is the only life I
have. The urgency for intravenous infusions of coherency presses
on our chest, bundles of bricks occluding breath. When was my
last expansive inhale? When was yours? Let's breathe softly in
synchrony, tuning our hearts to harmonic frequencies.

I quest wholeness,
not merely psychological empowerment.
What do you hunger for?
I am remarkably mortal—
a patchwork of flesh and bones that rip and tear at seams
    and simultaneously anti-fragile—
utterly uncertain as to the holding power of my
    endurance.
With this single breath, I intake the entire universe into
    my broken body. I am desperate to dance with painful
    memories, to unlock something secreted inside I never
    knew I contained, to break myself wide open until I am
    once again whole, to unleash a watershed of traumatic
    growth.
I am homesick for myself,
undeniably uncertain as to who I am at age 29,
a birthday that feels more like a death day.

I am exposed to a whole host of exotic elements. Ironically,
    life arises beneath the microscope of my attention,
    coming even closer to my consciousness the further
    my physical body becomes from the physical world.
    Disability narrows the gap between me and trees,
    between me and mountains, between me and turtles,
    between me and everything natural in this world.
All I have to do is reside in the still tide of my breath.

Do you know how to be in these blessed voids?
All I have to do is resist
resisting the cruel machinations of being.
I have become a remarkably strong tea,
verging on a bitter beverage—

I seep in thought,
drenching my neurons in looping contemplation
elicited by sheer isolation that grants me a type of vision I
    never knew existed,
I never wanted to receive.
And I wonder if words will ever be sufficient to hold me,
to capture my musings—
my loss,
my despair,
my itch to suffuse each moment with a dose of
    significance.
Perhaps words are more dependent on us to respire
than we on them in their callow
capacity to contain the uncontainable.
In my fear-drenched existence within the
empty spaces between these words,
I broach the fact
that I barely survived the unsurvivable
when I was nearly unhooked permanently from this world,
so all of my current fears must pale in comparison to that
    horror.
It is inescapably unclear as to whether there is a higher
    power in this world,
a master governor tensioning and slackening the strings.
But perhaps that concern is irrelevant to being here with
    this happening
I know better than to attempt to control.
Because I believe devoutly
not in overcoming,
not in resilience,
not in some creed,

but in the audacity to adapt as atoms drifting through
    space and time
that miraculously cohered into the person I was,
into the person I am evolving in this after the aftershock.
There is unraveling sadness here.
There is a floodgate of emergence from emergency.
There is the paradox of being human.
This stroke unzipped me from everything.
But I am learning that knowing and being are not
    synonymous.
Here I am-
a beautifully segmented 29-year-old girl
who is breathing through her grief,
parsing something approaching solace through tears—
water that yokes me to electric aliveness.

Second pruning

The first pruning tiptoes unnoticed, pruning itself as it
    manifests,
unhappening as it happens, in the foreground of our
    prelude,
a lineage we are excerpted from knowing, an Eden from
    which we are severed,
the mind burgeoning sparking circuits out of aimless seas
    of twitching networks,
entwining neurons firing without causality, too much
    noise for a signal to emerge—
our pre-analytical, pre-mathematical, pre-deductive,
    pre-reductive selves once upon a time fathomed so
    effortlessly the exotic artistry of just being-

a monolith of marble before Michelangelo's David chisels
   its way out of hiding.

We suddenly appear out of havoc, shapeless tendrils of
   wilderness diced into schemes
of homed organisms voracious to apprehend too much.

I have been canceled, separated from logic, didactics,
marked at the crown jewel of my cervical spine,
my nervous system decapitated, defeated, overthrown.

Throw evolution aside.

Toss self-determinism to the winds.

Hurl everything you ever deemed invincible in this world-
your very self- into the seas.
I am living evidence of hammer blows that strike us,
   disintegrate us
into microcosms of Darwinian principles unwriting
   themselves.

We can be minced within microseconds.

The gulf between my inclinations and my gated abilities is
   excruciating, menacing.

But the days, tell me how they click onwards, are yet my
   hammock.

Time punctuates my forehead with trembling trepidation,
and this heart gallops somewhere or nowhere, ignorant
of its residence or target.

I am distraught in the purposelessness of this hapless slant
   of being.

These spoken bites of tear-choked crackling sound uncurl
    on my tongue-
a limp object the right half of which bewilders my brain.

I lack structure, so I impose it on these lines.

My uncharted right borders
fly wide open, declaring me more infinite, spectral, one
    with this
uncreated world that neither ends nor begins.

I am lost, foregone and forgotten as an individual.

This verse- a snapshot of a life in
perpetual flight,
distressingly out of date.

There is nothing neutral about disability.

We shuffle words about to frame narrative,
lacing the portrait we lack brushes to paint with syllabic
    pearls
chinked with essential emptiness that enlivens the faulty
documents of our bodies with the scent of wings.

We define and remake ourselves with galaxies of
language rippling with starlight that floods us even
when the floodgates of our bodies,
the floorboards on which we stand,
are far beyond shores of reform.

I cannot be replenished of self.

If only.

I cannot be unpruned of this stroke.

I repel, without a harness, off the cliffside
of self, precipitously landing on the foggy white
abyss of loss as it furrows its way into me,
ensnaring me in chasms between these words.

I am pruned back-
the umbilical cord snapped between
me and reality,
an aggrieved misstep.

I am pain raging,
a process unprocessing,
mournfully late to my own future as it turns its neck
and scampers off in the opposite direction,
leaving me stitched into the distressing truth of
my own brokenness,
my entire universe
pruned by a singular synapse
cut by a doctor's blade.

The singe of a needle
permeating the threshold
of my body pruned me
of everything.

I am an empty vessel stuck at the base
of a black hole no one else even knows about.

I am out of bounds of neuroscience,
of knowledge of myself, in the garbled din of
surreal silence of disability.

I am a tree.
I shed my leaves.

Find me the shape of honor in this
second pruning of disability.

I am fumbling in fumes of thick pale air that leave me
    wheezing,
panting for oxygen to return my breath to my body,
my mind pruned of perspective,
deserted in the mud of incoherent limbs out of tune
with each other, flapping about as though they were
never intended to be wedded into the same united front.

You do not get a day,
a moment,
off from disability.

We cannot even swing a speck of holidays that do not
unscramble their way
into sense anymore in this upside-down
filled to the neck with overwhelm.

My brain is dislodged—
the sensory map of my right half
shredded.

Let me know if you locate my belongings.

I am wrong, loose in the socket of my stroke.

The word progress unmoors me from
whatever scant bearings linger here.

Oh, my besmirched fall from
my body's graces.

I am now tangential to myself,
a respiring non-sequitur.

If only this anarchy,
this ceaseless winter solstice,
could yield to spring.

I am an icon of pathless agony.

Oh, the
heights from which we can
fall that give way to
ample and unspoken terrors.

The neurons that wire me into
this minute no longer entice me-
their transmitter choreography
no longer terrain I effervesce to know.

Involuntarily,
I missed my own peak.

But innocence never abandons us.
We give it away, throw our hands upward,
repelled by the propulsive indignity
of the universe,
the flames it casts our way, entropy darting itself at the
    very
pavement you ached to pave,
vanished, washed out.

We are chalk on gravel.

Beware of rain.

Maybe I can enchant my remaining nerves into firing the
circuitry of hope, a smile writing itself
on a mouth that remembers taste.

I want to run away from this ongoing
infestation of my life.

But, beneath this unbearable smog of grief,
I know I will, one day,
find a million and one pixels-
that there is far more to my story, to me, to you, to us
then I currently know.

Reunion

I glance in bafflement at photographs taken behind the
    wrought iron bars
of my before, flabbergasted by the person beaming who is
    both me and not me—
someone bursting with luminous vitality, at once a refugee
    and a familiar acquaintance.

Her smile looks like a summer sky ignited with fireworks,
lighting up her entire being,
as though she were a fluorescent jellyfish on the ocean
    floor, an emblem of elation,
something elevated above the level of words, above the
    realm of conscious thought.

She, like the right side of my body in this epilogue, is an
    absent presence, a shadowy creature from a dreamy
    planet, another genre of existence, who feels as though
    she emanates from fictional passages, from utopian
    corridors of imagination.

She seems to patronize my now mangled body from her
    lofty joyous wholeness.

The parts of me still intact are enraged that she and I were
   once synonymous.

I desire the simplicity of a delete key to appear within my
   hippocampus,
to cut her out,
so she no longer captivates my psyche, so she no longer
   haunts me with lugubrious loss that leaves me panting
   and
feeling as though I belong beneath the Earth if the
soles of my feet can no longer tread upon it with sensory
   ease.

She used to dance for no reason without music as she
   selected her shirt each morning.

She used to wander without a destination through
   sidewalks parched for words present in poetry she
   carried in her hands and palpability pressed into her soul.

She smiled at the world as it spun on its axis before her
   eyes,
as spring transitioned into summer,
as flowers ruptured into being, as birds festooned the sky,
   as ants and ladybugs skittered across her bare arms and
   feet.

How can I be that person?

Permit me to pause for a moment to register this grief-
this annihilation of feeling from the right
part of my body, from my mind annexed in darkness.

Show me the path homeward.

Is there such a path?

I need another moment, another series of breaths. I do not
    have the words yet.

Maybe I do not always need the words I presume I need.

Maybe I need to live the truth, rather than express it in
    blunt black and white.

I want to grant myself the gentle kindness to be changed
    by this trauma.

I want to grant myself the ability to learn without needing
to preserve that learning in language,
but rather to feel it in my body.

I have forgotten what a smile feels like—
how it stretches and tugs at the corners of the mouth,
how it simultaneously contracts and expands the capacity
    to see-
squinting the outward gaze while thrusting open a
    different type of vision-
how it creases the forehead with temporary tattoos of
    delight,
how it changes your entire world because
it changes you from inside out.

Though I long for her innocence
I struggle to call my own to evaporate,
I also thirst for her to appear in my after,
if only for a jaunt,
if only to murmur in my left ear-
the only functional ear I have left—

that she and I may have another chance,
an opportunity for a reunion.

Though I mourn her, tears flooding my entire being,
with a degree or two of hostility,
with a double dose of disillusioned disbelief,
I am terrified of trampling upon her,
of translating her out of comprehension,
of extracting her as though she were but an organ
    prepared for transplantation.

Wherever she continues to linger on in some limbo within,
I will permit her to persist.

As I select these words, a thunderstorm of tears rings
    through me.

I have come to realize that she encapsulates all that was
    lost,
all that was swiftly stolen,
when the mortal shell of my being
was cracked wide open,
ransacking me of myself.

I sense her jerky and reticent crawl towards me.

I extend my arms—
both the one I can feel and the one I can no longer feel—
outwards in her direction,
reaching myself through time,
into the improbable and the possible,
into anyone I once was or can now become.

"Thrownness"

Heidegger's ripening of the sharp spear of a verb into a
    descriptor,
sound that thrusts its way, banging between your tongue
    and the roof of
your mouth, hammer blows of sonic verbal chaos
    emulating connotation,
ontology of being, mortality thrown, paintballs exploding,
colliding into circumstance beyond bounds of choice,
into communion with the world, stapled into situations,
desperate for harbingers that never arrive,
prescriptions expurgated from the eternal pandemic of
    mortality.

Being human is no alphabetized, orderly condition—
there is no library,
no librarian,
no book-shelving to bind us into refuge of illusions we
    fruitlessly desire.

We are too friable,
too breakable, too thrown against thrownness.

Thrownness—
we cannot usurp nor shuffle past this reality.

We are slots defined by our own emptiness, negative
    spaces—
we cannot return the texts of ourselves, however many
    lacunae preside.

Thrownness—
we are smashed out of paradise by the thunderstorm of
    thrownness.

Thrownness—
we cannot negotiate with you.

We are evasive, lurking around the bend from ourselves,
    zip-lines of flesh
casting their way, gambling in the trembling whiplash of
    the world.

No anarchy of language,
no matter the jab, the jaggedness
of words, will overthrow thrownness.

We must peel our eyes from screens, from our technology-
    obsessed shellacked shells.

We are no snow globes in consistently spinning worlds.

We are breakable, on the pockmarked landscape
of the universe too fractured and fracturable—
two worlds meeting, a temporary conversation we mistake
    for
unblemished permanence impermeable to thrownness.

Thrownness—
we exist on the perimeter of ourselves,
cows grazing outskirts of fields,
neglecting the racing evergreen heart at the center.

The random, askance universe does not catch us.

Thrownness—
the fork of my maimed spinal cord, a crude dissection of
    memory between
past and present, before and after-
I reside in the spectrum,
in between, somewhere orthogonal to the here and now,
on bridges we construct through thrownness as we rescue
    but cannot unbreak ourselves.

Oh, how words pull me into their gravity, animating me
    with movement.

We contuse ourselves with too much information,
    exhausting wattage of mind,
labeling it stress, efficiency, purpose.

We concentrate too much—
limit our wings of attention to minutia, bated and battered
    by too much
thinking.

Fear, a second skin that clings, clots breath.

I am a raw nerve, exposed to the elements,
thrown into vigilance, awash in the tide of pain that
    disorders thoughts, offers nowhere to turn as my body
    betrays me,
thwarting, twisting space and time,
disintegrating discussions of
weather,
highlights,
nail polish,
made up portraits of faces,
fancy sandwiches,

chai lattes,
appearances,
clothing,
the boundary layer of existence,
routine, ritual,
dishwashers into
cacophonous hodgepodge of syllables when your borders
     have been knifed,
your life at 27 thrown into palimpsests of conflict,
     catastrophe and contradiction,
your life now crippled, curtailed.

We are all lost in space until we lose space-
that is precisely when we are found.

Thrownness—
tomorrow is not promised.

The interface between me and my numb right side—
a foot bridge, a narrow corridor straining to be eyed.

Thrownness—
we cannot coax our way out the entropy- the angelic and
     the horrific that zap us all.

Are you scared of darkness' advent?

Let's outgrow lament together in tandem with words that
     poke at what we
aim to distend with language but are not armed with the
     right dialect,
the right glances and expressions that worm their way into
     our souls.

We are all but a minute shy of dependence, growing
into the holes that thread us through into the thrownness
   of humanity.

Loss is a quarry of rocks,
but we are but are but feathers.

Thrownness—
we are hollow.

Thrownness—
we are replete.

All Is contingent on the screw of parallax,
the dial of perspective.

Thrownness—
I need hope to be a denser thing, not a flimsy word,
but my father's sturdy shoulders on which I can perch
   without falling.

Thrownness—
a minute passes, a decade, a life.

Thrownness—
is there a warranty for a life, a buffer against our meekness?

We are not durable things.

We are interdependent organisms, rhizomes on roots.
We are in dialectical tension with ourselves.

Shield me against this ghostly draft of self as she is
   triggered,
unwittingly, from the dentist's chair—
the gauntlet of her right arm aspiring to be

a skyscraper,
a massive mass swinging on the pendulum of the cosmos,
the blaring scream of the hygienist's electric tool in the
   way
of her arm's flight attempt,
a dancing spree,
a tango through the cloud of air that hits the screen
of an elbow,
the tool aloft,
the noise vanishing,
as my eyes locate my arm.

How loud the thundering articulation of my limb, ripping
   through
the syncopated instrument, the exuberant
ruckus of motion coughing in starts and fits.

I nuzzle this numb extremity within the left hand I still
   have
left to feel, a restraining order against the desecrated right
   side,
a strange cocktail of absurdity, outrage and grief, making
   its way to the base of my throat.

Thrownness—
how quickly we are shorn of the armament of our bodies
   that unspool in the squint of a pinch of a minute.

Thrownness—
we are unmonitored wildlife.

Let us respect the influx of our fledgling bodies,
our souls that keep reaching for radiance,

for light, no matter the lack of a dimmer switch on our
    blackouts,
earthquakes that rumble through our bodies at all once,
or over the slow spillage of time slipping through soil.

Thrownness—
bless my right side that misremembers me.
How I quest to cull you into me, a lullaby of touch.

Thrownness—
there is no class you can cut, no truancy for the human
    condition—
precarious,
terrible,
awesome.

Oh, the vertiginous drop of flesh against the floor of
    thrownness—
my autonomy atomized.

We do not test our own gravity, a force that tests us.
We skirt under it and around it, hiding until it finds us,
    debris in the defunct
cul-de-sac of the world, until we catch our breath,
    recognize
the precipice from which we fell can also be a door,
another self in relief against the ruins of what was, a
    treasured texture of brush strokes sealed behind the
    surface of another painting.

Thrownness—
my discharge from intensive care, from life support,
did not discharge me from trauma, from the disturbance
    of disability,

from brainstem damage fencing you into a body you
  deem laced
with shame- the ticking of judgment winding through
  your mind, a thunderclap disassembling you, muting,
  dulling, my essence, our inescapable thrownness.

Right side,
I do not want to reject and resist you anymore.

Thrownness—
my leaky boundary on my right half,
this tortured loss transfiguring the topography of my
  being is
morphing into a vista, an opening in the torn tent of my
  body, a refined sense of
becoming my own guardian, infusing me with awareness
  of being alive-
a coming into still quiet, a coming home to an inner grace.

I do not need a neatly ordered, unencumbered spinal cord
  to feel.

Do you?

I no longer need to wear to fear on my nervous system
  through each minute.

I am ever so slowly learning my body never left me but
  was here the whole time.

Do you know how to listen to your body in staggering
  silence?

Thrownness—
bless this plodding industry of growing a soul,

of learning to not be mortified by your vulnerable
nervous system seething in aftershocks,
the heaps of you you do not know what to do with,
a hand of cards without a home of the remainder of the
   deck,
because the rug was snatched beneath your feet and you
   slid
somewhere at the bottom of the ocean, washing you
   away, or so you presumed, but you are still here—
diffident, different, distorted,
but here resoundingly,
undeniably, staunchly, devoutly mortal.

I am united- a pioneer on the frontier of self—
searching, squinting,
squirming, redacted,
rewritten, remade.

Thrownness—
universe, throw me back into innocence again- into wind
   whisking,
ruffling my downy mop of curls.

The pastel of time knows us all.

Thrownness—
I clothe myself in questions, imponderables niggling at the
   corners of your mind, lodged in my right side, phones off
   the hook ringing, music only met with hearing,
not a calculator, not a solution set, not bile of fear,
but a with a newfangled, unarticulated form of trust
creaking through the universe, a revelation of senses lost
   and earned.

I write to return myself back to myself.

I am here
to cry, to laugh,
to feel the pain, the pause, the paucity,
the beautiful, the incredible
brokenness of being human.

Thrownness—
I cohere to myself without coherence—
no textbook nor how-to guides can dictate nor direct
    existence.

Let's let time pass through us, around us, without
    perforating
shock zapping through us in anxiety and terror at what we
    have become—
these unalterably, remarkably
shattered organisms relentlessly gathering whatever shafts
    of light
wander through our night—
this is where we shake hands with ourselves.

Are you ready to sink with me into the preverbal preface of
    beginning again?

Permit us to let our disgruntled bodies be exactly as they
    are.

Let's land here- palms facing upwards,
receiving the thrownness that links us to nothing and
    everything at once.

Thrownness—
bless the capacity, however constrained, to occupy space,
　to re-pose
over and again, to come into the shimmering contagion of
　belonging with others,
with our altered configurations, as we brazenly assume
prayer pose, mountain pose, warrior pose—
the current and currency of the body,
even mine on the solemn shorelines of my naïveté stroke.

Bless us as we lengthen from the crown of our head to our
　tailbone,
the unstructured equation and equilibrium of my body
　offset, but not dead.

Thrownness—
I know how to feel time, let an exhale dilate in me,
the mechanistic bleeping soundscape of the intensive
　care ward my teacher.

I need to begin reciprocating love to this body, this flimsy,
　undone,
spine that can no longer envelope all of me.

But there is so much more to having a body
than purely having a physically intact body.

Thrownness—
we are all astronauts, floating passengers adrift in
　thrownness.

My disabled right side instructs my able left.

We dispute, protest as we descend into anachronisms,
　incompletion, obsolescence,

lurching into sadness without any railing to break our
    thrownness.

Thrownness—
just as suddenly and stupefyingly as we
are unmade, my mother's unfalteringly loving glance is
    coupled with
terms of endearment- lovey or honey- shock-absorbers in
    the shape
of sugary monikers that waft through my body,
a cotton candy I can taste in more in my disabled than in
    my
able body, a hug slicing despair, notes suspended in the
    hammock of silence,
reverberating, a chorus line that loops endlessly on itself
in the record player of my soul.

I am held.

I am worthy.

I am cherished.

You are too.

Thrownness—
bless these syllables in the frozen climate of my soul.

For even once they hit the boiling point of flight into silent
    molecules hissing through air, they are stuck in me, in
    the ember of my spirit,
tender warm light thrown into my wintering within walls
    where music has an
afterlife long after it yields to the thrownness of everything.

Bless us as we come undone and heroically remake our
    way,
interdigitating ourselves into the flock of humanity,
the ties that bind us into who we always were.

Thrownness—
bless the courage that we welcome as it peruses our
    askance forms.

Bless us for feeling the weak drizzle of gratitude,
even when our lives feel revoked.

Our souls surge, our bodies recalibrate, becoming abodes
    of a million
and one emotions.

Thrownness—
bless us for blessing ourselves as we emerge into being
    outside of
context and categories, leaning towards each other as we
    awaken
from the coma of trauma.

We feel everything.

We see all and continue to smile when we are shaken with
    compassion.

Here is my hand.

Permit me to gently take yours.

Thrownness—
bless the slack tension of our stray days.

Bless us as we come unknotted—

shoelaces flustered in the breeze, as we are impeached
  from ourselves,
forced to shed the skin of our becoming, but continue to
  laugh, to emerge from our own erasure, to smile at the
  sheer fact of our endurance, of our somber continuity,
as we begin to view loss as a prism, not a prison,
but a lens into an opening we never before saw.

Anointed

I recolor my way outside linear narrative,
reverse gears out of platonic ideals life never quite adopts
into sublime coupling.

I am half doubled,
a revised, reseen poem
polishing itself new.

Ayurvedic oils modulate out of phase waveforms cresting
through my clattering dissonant
call and response.

I am cynical, crass,
peripatetic, incorrigible,
a lost continent drifting away from Pangea.

I no longer strive to accomplish the impossible-
to hive myself off, to pass as though I have been unaddled
  by circumstance—
but to let go into family long awaiting my advent into
  disability.

I pain to be unmarked by the commensurate volume of
  wonder deflated,

because life is shoring up dazzling meaning
as people flattened by tragedy's collateral reseed
dimension in tandem with my second adolescence.

My brain slackens to bind and bandage myself with
    empiricism,
boiling pots cradling themselves to calmer seas.

I placidly settle off-kilter.

I am anointed into the kingdom of my unwinding self
as embers marry my able and disabled composites—
tuning forks transforming formless din into a Stradivarius
    violin,
a euphonious chord you play on strings of my stanzas,
sanctifying me as you scan these syllables.

I pick up this brand-new baton the universe tosses my
    way.

I crackle into awakening into someone
I effortlessly love in all of her complex beauty.

I am coalescing into formation,
an unaddressed incarnation flowers,
concretizing me into someone I cherish,
someone worth evolving.

I peel away from running away,
from churning my faltering body into a house of horrors.

I am twisting darkness into a fumbling spring I regenerate
    within.

My growl is editing itself into a subtle smile.
My thumping heart catches its breath.

I am born of the womb of sorrow kindred with hope,
budding from the pit of trauma.

I am transcendent—
a flint of bioluminescence,
the aurora borealis articulating its bold
evanescent brushstrokes across the canvas of night.

This shadowland turns out to be a wonderland.

I am my own bride.

Conclusion

In her verses, the speaker alchemizes the synapses pruned from her central nervous system, seas of silence, language's absences, and even the word "disability" into reservoirs of potential energy. At the close of this section, the speaker unlocks a sense of anointment into this life, a beckoning into who she is becoming and a desire to greet this nascent version of herself with rising belief. She is empowered. She is light.

Conclusion

The experience of suffering a stroke alters a person's life, often cruelly. In the aftermath of Elly's hospitalization, being bedridden and unable to find solace in the science and math that had been her bedrock, dispossession took over and a veil of silence settled over her. Neither higher education nor daily vigilance gave her any refuge from what her life had become, and grief's waves crashed against what no longer was, stapling her mouth shut. She distrusted her own faculties and was haunted by what in her life hadn't happened, and by what had. Nearly a year of silence passed before she desired to shape words around her wound, and she realized the power of dictation.

As soon as she began dictating her thoughts, Elly had unlocked the mechanism that saves her life each day from the onslaught of her disability. At first, she could only compose one fugitive fragment a day, in light of her stroke's breaks on her cognition and intermittent aphasia. Sometimes, language surged at high-tide. At other times, words halted. The accident of discovering the power of poetry to express herself happening concurrently with her stroke continues to serve as a medium for self-evolution and resurrection, a shield she leverages at dawn to compose suffering into song.

Acknowledgments

Part 1 Overture was published in the *San Antonio Review*, December 2024.

Discussion questions

1. How does the speaker evolve throughout this section?
2. How does using different pronouns serve as a means to cope with trauma?
3. What role does memory play as her narrative unfolds?
4. In what ways does writing itself shift the speaker's sense of self and the impression of disability on her changing identity?
5. How do her relationships, to others and to writing, help return the speaker's viewpoint to the first person?

Recommended readings

Blevins, Alison, *Cataloguing Pain,* YesYes Books, 2023.

Blevins, Alison, *Handbook for the Newly Disabled*, Blazevox, 2022.

Judd, Bettina, *Patient. Poems,* Black Lawrence Press, 2014.

Robson, Ruthann, *Notes on my Dying*, Creative Nonfiction, Issue 18, 2001.

Williams, Wendy Patrice, *Autobiography of a Sea Creature: Healing the Trauma of Infant Surgery*, UC Health Humanities Press, 2023.

A Body You Talk To: An Anthology of Contemporary Disability, edited by Tennison S. Black, Sundress Publications, 2023.

In Between Spaces, *An Anthology of Disabled Writers*, edited by Rebecca Burke, Stillhouse Press, 2022.

Index

* 9 781917 503334 *